Dr David Chadwick, DM, Fl̲~~~~~~~~~~~~~~~
ogy at the University of ~~~~~~~~~~~~~~~~~
Hospital, Liverpool, where ~~~~~~ ~~ ~~~~~ ~ ~~~~~~
clinic for people with epilepsy. He is also involved in
research on the effects of drug treatment, which takes
him to many other epilepsy centres worldwide. He is
married with two children.

Sue Usiskin has had epilepsy for more than 30 years.
She is a counsellor at the National Hospital, London,
where since 1989 she has offered a dedicated service to
people with epilepsy and their families.

She also speaks widely on the pscho-social aspects of
living with epilepsy to physicians, nurses, carers and
schools. She has contributed to many publications and
media productions and in 1995 won the Ambassador for
Epilepsy award. She is married with two children.

LIVING WITH
EPILESPY

A practical guide to coping, causes and treatment

Dr David Chadwick
and
Sue Usiskin

Diagrams by
Kevin Marks

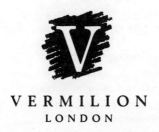

VERMILION
LONDON

First published in Great Britain in 1987 by Macdonald Optima
Revised edition published by Optima in 1991.

1 3 5 7 9 10 8 6 4 2

This edition published in the United Kingdom in 1997 by Vermilion, an
imprint of Ebury Press
Random House UK
Random House
20 Vauxhall Bridge Road
London SW1V 2SA

Random House Australia (Pty) Ltd
20 Alfred Street
Milsons Point
Sydney
New South Wales 2016 Australia

Random House New Zealand Limited
18 Poland Road, Glenfield
Auckland 10 New Zealand

Random House South Africa (Pty) Ltd
Endulini, 5A Jubilee Road
Parktown 2193, South Africa

Random House UK Limited Reg. No 954009
A CIP catalogue record for this book is available from the British
Library

ISBN: 0 09 181431 7

Typeset in Palatino by Deltatype Ltd, Birkenhead, Merseyside
Printed and bound in Great Britain by Mackays of Chatham, plc

Papers used by Vermilion are natural, recyclable products made from
wood grown in sustainable forests.

*I dedicate this book to the memory of my mother,
who taught me what courage was, and to
my husband Andrew and children Oliver and
Anna for their love, support and humour.*   SU

CONTENTS

ACKNOWLEDGMENTS

I thank all my patients with epilepsy, without whose help this book would never have been written. I should also like to thank Mr Peter Rogan for his help and advice on schooling and epilepsy.   DC

I thank Professor Simon Shorvon for the opportunity to counsel his patients from whom I have learnt very much. I also thank Dr Michael Isaac for his helpful supervision of my work and Susan Voss who typed my manuscript.   SU

PREFACE

Epilepsy is a common condition that affects millions of people, yet no disorder can claim to be as misunderstood. While heart attacks and even cancer can be discussed openly and frankly today, epilepsy is a subject that is rarely talked about, and one that still carries a considerable social stigma. The reasons for this are understandable. To observers, epileptic seizures can be frightening, confusing, and even violent occurrences, during which people who are outwardly identical to themselves suddenly lose consciousness. They might fall to the floor, possibly injuring themselves and becoming incontinent. The reluctance to discuss the condition perpetuates the misunderstanding, which adds to the burden of epilepsy. This means that people with epilepsy often have to cope not only with their disorder, but also with problems making friends, and making progress at school and at work.

Around 2–3 percent of the population have recurrent epileptic seizures at some time in their lives, so many people have a friend or relative with the condition. At some time you may witness an epileptic seizure, in the street, in a store or at a big gathering. Everyone should know what this looks like and be able to give the right assistance. Equipped with the proper information, people are less likely to be hostile to epilepsy.

In this book we aim to provide a basic understanding of epilepsy for people with the condition, their families and anyone who has regular contact with them. The information and advice given here will help dispel the myths and misconceptions about epilepsy, and allow people to make commonsense decisions about their everyday lives and activities. We shall show how in spite of epilepsy it is possible to lead an active, enjoyable and relatively unrestricted life.

Section I

What Is Epilepsy?

1

What is epilepsy?

Epilepsy has affected people for as long as history has been recorded. The term is derived from a Greek word that means 'to take hold of, to seize or to possess'. Although this reflects the ancient Greeks' belief that an epileptic attack represented possession by the gods, by about 400 BC the Hippocratic writers identified epilepsy as a physical disorder of the brain and pointed out that damage to one side of the brain can lead to convulsions that affect mainly the opposite side of the body. It was defined by the British neurologist Hughlings Jackson a century ago as a recurrent, episodic, uncontrolled discharge of nerve tissue.

How many people have epilepsy?

It is difficult to be certain, but it seems that between two and three in every 100 members of the population have recurrent seizures at some time in their lives. Fortunately, the majority of these people do not have epilepsy throughout their lives. The chart overleaf shows the age-related incidence and prevalence of epilepsy. Incidence is the number of people developing epilepsy for the first time during each year, that is, the number of new cases. Prevalence refers to the number of people who have the disorder in any given year; in other words, all new cases plus existing ones. You can see that epilepsy develops most often during the first 10 to 20 years of life. Many people developing it at this time do not have seizures during later life. However, some people do go on suffering from the condition for longer periods, and this, taken with the fact that epilepsy develops at a lesser rate in the later years of life, means that prevalence increases with age.

Epileptic seizures and epilepsy

An epileptic attack, or seizure, is a relatively brief episode of altered behaviour or consciousness that has a rapid beginning, is usually short and self-limiting, and might be followed by a period of drowsiness and confusion. There are many different types of seizure and it is important to realize that anyone can have a seizure given the appropriate circumstances. It is the way a normal brain responds to a number of abnormal conditions. For example, someone who develops an infection of the brain – such as meningitis, encephalitis or a brain abscess – or who has liver or kidney failure, or who takes an excess of any one of a number of drugs, including alcohol, can have one or more seizures. Although such a person might have recurrent seizures due to such a condition, he or she is not thought of as having epilepsy, because the liability to seizures will end when the underlying condition is cured.

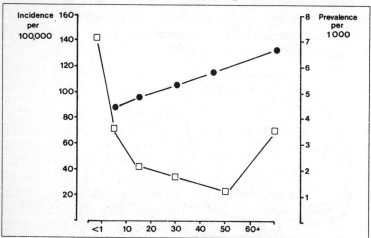

The incidence and prevalence of epilepsy at different ages.

Epilepsy is a condition in which seizures recur, usually spontaneously. It is a disorder of the function of the brain itself, which sometimes results from the scarring of, or other damage to, the brain. So while we all can potentially have seizures, fewer people have epilepsy. To understand the nature of epilepsy, we need to understand the structure and function of the normal brain.

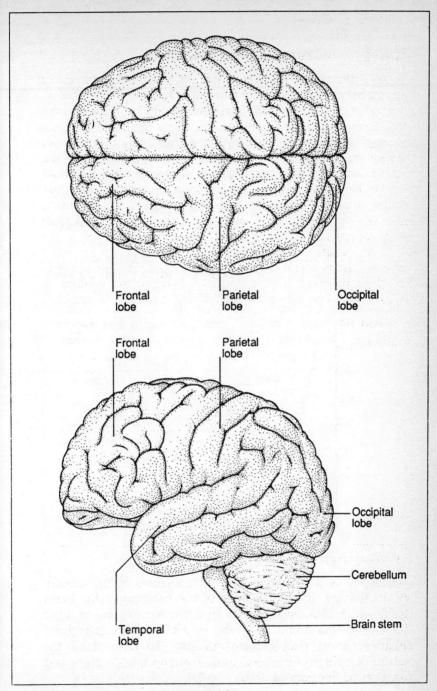

Frontal lobe
Parietal lobe
Occipital lobe

Frontal lobe
Parietal lobe

Occipital lobe

Cerebellum

Brain stem

Temporal lobe

The brain pictured from above and from the left.

How the brain works

The human brain consists of two cerebral hemispheres with connecting tracts that run through the brain stem into the spinal cord. The cerebral hemispheres contain large numbers of nerve cells, called neurons, which are responsible for our understanding and perception of the world about us, as well as for the control of our movements and emotions. The nerve cells are interconnected in a vast and infinitely complicated network, and each one can receive messages from hundreds of other cells and send messages to hundreds more.

Nerve cells communicate with each other by electrical means. When a nerve cell is activated, or fired, an electrical current runs along the nerve fibre and releases a chemical substance, called a neurotransmitter, at the points, or synapses, where it touches other cells. The neurotransmitters can either excite the second cell or inhibit it. If it is sufficiently excited, the second cell will fire, discharging its neurotransmitter to connect with and influence other cells. However, if the second cell receives an inhibitory signal, it will not fire. In

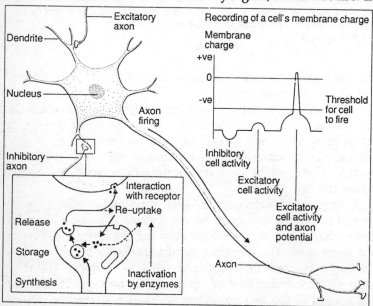

The ways in which nerve cells (neurons) influence each other and their firing.

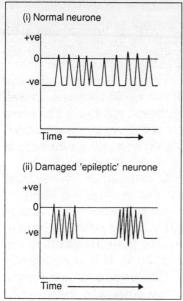

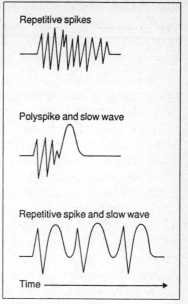

The patterns of activity that can be recorded from (i) a normal cell and (ii) a cell that has been damaged to make it 'epileptic'.

Different types of EEG abnormalities that can be seen in epilepsy.

this way information is transmitted, integrated and filtered within our nervous system.

A normal nerve cell tends to fire repetitively at a relatively low frequency. If the cell is made epileptic by being damaged, its pattern of firing changes. Instead of discharging at low frequencies, it discharges at extremely high frequencies in bursts. There might be long periods between these bursts when the cell is inactive.

A single cell behaving in this abnormal, epileptic way would not cause anyone to have a seizure. A seizure happens only when many thousands of cells behave in this fashion at the same time. The resulting disturbance may be reflected in the first symptoms of an epileptic seizure – its aura – and may then alter the behaviour of other normal nerve cells, causing the spread of the seizure. When we use an electroencephalogram (EEG) to record changes in the electrical activity, we find that the sudden discharge of several thousand nerve cells usually results in 'spikes' and these are sometimes followed by a slow wave of reduced activity *(see figure on page 7).*

Now that we know how an epileptic seizure begins in the brain, we can look at how it affects people.

2

Types of epileptic seizure

We have seen that a basic abnormality in the function of the nerve cells in the brain leads to a seizure. The brain is so complex that very similar abnormalities in its different areas will produce very different effects in different people. This means that there is an enormous variety of seizures – there probably are as many different kinds of seizure as there are people having them. In spite of this we have to attempt to classify the seizures broadly, because different kinds of seizure can carry very different outlooks (prognoses), have different implications and require different treatment.

A simplified classification of seizures is shown in the table on page 10. The major differentiation is between:

● seizures that begin in a localized part of the brain and usually spread slowly, which we call partial or focal seizures, and
● seizures that affect the whole of both cerebral hemispheres from very early in the seizure, which we call generalized seizures

We can usually differentiate between these two kinds of seizures on the basis of what a person experiences before and afterwards, and, perhaps most important, from the description by someone who was there at the time. An EEG can give us further information *(see pages 48–51)*.

Partial seizures

Partial, or focal, seizures begin in a restricted part of one of the cerebral hemispheres. When a seizure discharge begins in this way, the remaining parts of both cerebral hemispheres continue to work normally. The person is conscious but experiences a number of abnormal symptoms, reflecting the normal working of the part of the brain that is affected. This is the warning, or aura, of an epileptic seizure. All attacks of this kind can spread from the site of onset to involve other parts of the brain. In this way both hemispheres can become affected and a generalized seizure can occur. After a partial seizure is over, symptoms might persist and they again reflect the part of the brain where the seizure began. The EEGs of people with partial seizures often show that any electrical abnormalities between seizures affect only a particular area of one of the cerebral hemispheres.

Classification of Seizures

Partial seizures (begin locally)

Simple: consciousness not impaired
   a. with motor symptoms
   b. with somatosensory or special sensory symptoms
   c. with autonomic symptoms
   d. with psychic symptoms

Complex: consciousness impaired
   a. beginning as a simple partial seizure and progressing to a complex seizure
   b. impairment of consciousness at onset
      i. impairment of consciousness only
      ii. with automatism
Partial seizures that become generalized (to tonic-clonic seizures)

Generalized seizures

Absence seizures
   a. simple (petit mal)
   b. complex
Myoclonic seizures

Clonic seizures

Tonic seizures

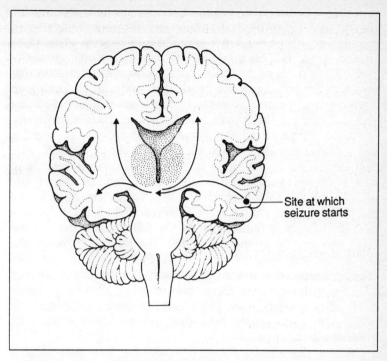

The onset of a partial seizure in the temporal lobe and the pathways by which it can spread to cause a generalized seizure.

Tonic-clonic seizures

Atonic seizures

What can happen to people during a partial seizure? Let us first consider the partial seizures that are called simple seizures.

Motor seizures

The frontal lobe of each hemisphere controls movement of the opposite side of the body. Therefore, when a seizure begins in the left frontal lobe, movement is produced on the right side of the body, and vice versa. This usually results in what is called an aversive seizure, which affects mainly the head, eyes and arms. In the tonic phase of the seizure *(see page 18)* the person feels his or her head and eyes being drawn irresistibly to one side; his or her hand or arm might become stiff and be drawn upwards. This might be followed by a clonic phase *(see page 18)*, periods of muscular contraction and relaxation that result in the jerking of the head, arm, and leg. Following an aversive fit, people sometimes experience a short-lasting weakness or paralysis, which is known as Todd's paralysis.

Another type of motor attack is the Jacksonian seizure, named after the British neurologist Hughlings Jackson, who first described it. Although it is rare, it is worth describing here because it shows how seizures can spread from their site of onset. A Jacksonian attack can begin with jerking affecting the thumb of one hand. As the fit spreads, the jerking spreads first to the whole hand, then to the whole arm, then to the face, and finally to the leg. When the jerking involves the whole of one side of the body, the person might lose consciousness and have a typical tonic-clonic seizure *(see page 18)*. If you look at the illustration on page 13, which shows how different parts of the frontal lobe relate to the parts of the body, you can picture how this seizure spreads from its original site of onset.

One of the frontal lobes (usually the left one) is also concerned with producing speech, and sudden 'speech arrest' sometimes occurs during a frontal lobe seizure. Between 20 and 30 per cent of people with partial seizures have seizures starting in the frontal lobes.

Sensory seizures

The parietal lobe is concerned with physical sensations. When a seizure starts in one of the parietal lobes, a person first feels a tingling, warmth or other peculiar sensation in a part of the opposite side of the body. Because the part of the parietal lobe that deals with sensation, say in the hand, is intimately connected with the part of the frontal lobe that moves that part of the body, it is quite common for seizures that begin with a sensation also to result in movement. In the same way that motor seizures can be followed by a period of apparent paralysis, sensory seizures can be followed by a period of numbness. Seizures starting in the parietal lobe are rare.

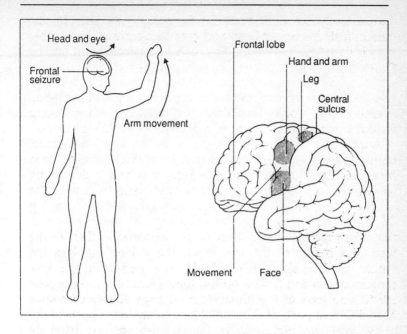

A simple partial seizure arising in the right frontal lobe. The picture of the brain shows which parts of the frontal lobe move which parts of the opposite side of the body.

Visual seizures

The occipital lobe at the back of the brain deals with vision. If a seizure begins in this part of the brain, a person experiences abnormal vision, which can be in the form of flashing lights, balls of light or complicated colours. As in the other types of seizure described above, the experience occurs on the side of the body – in this case, the visual field – opposite to the lobe where the seizure begins.

Simple seizures and the temporal lobe

The temporal lobe is a very common site for the origin of epileptic seizures. Unlike the frontal, parietal and occipital lobes, which have single clearly defined functions in terms of moving, feeling or seeing, the temporal lobe has many

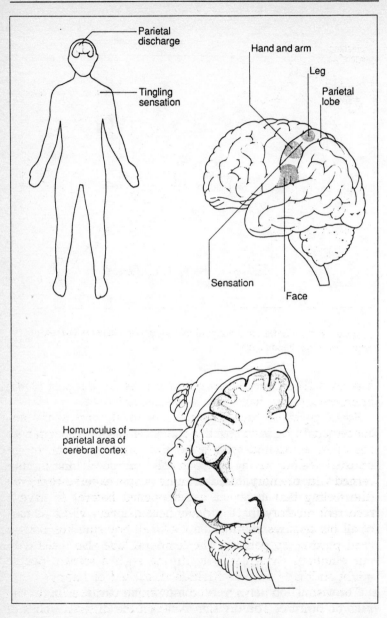

A simple sensory seizure arising in the right parietal lobe and causing abnormal sensations on the opposite side of the body.

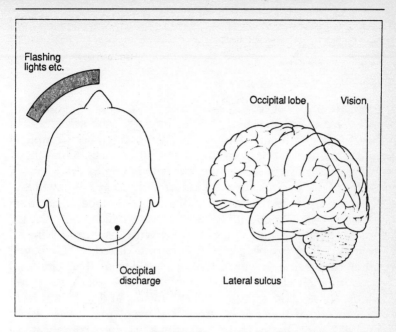

A seizure arising in the right occipital lobe. Abnormal visual sensations are perceived to the person's left.

functions. Therefore, when seizures arise in this part of the brain, people can have very varied experiences.

Some parts of the temporal lobe deal with sensations concerned with eating. For this reason seizures that begin here are often associated with a peculiar smell or taste, or an unusual feeling in the stomach. The temporal lobe is concerned with memory, too, and some people experience *déjà vu* (the feeling that an event has happened before) or have a recurrent memory that suddenly becomes very vivid; as part of all his seizures one man saw a small boy running along a road picking up pennies. The temporal lobe also deals with our emotions, which is why during such a seizure people might suddenly become frightened, excited or happy.

The distinction between all these simple partial seizures can become blurred. The division between the different lobes of the brain is somewhat artificial and some seizures that start in the parietal lobe with a sensory disturbance will, for example, spread to the temporal lobe so that the person may experience a combination of symptoms.

Complex partial seizures

These are the most common kinds of partial seizure and in the past were called psychomotor or temporal lobe seizures, as they most commonly arise in the temporal lobe. Complex partial seizures differ from simple partial seizures in that they are associated with some alteration in consciousness.

Often they begin with the kind of symptoms we have just described for seizures arising in the temporal lobe. Later, the person appears to go into a trance during which he or she is remote, detached and out of contact with his surroundings. He may fall. Some people simply appear dazed; others have rather confused behaviour, perhaps picking at their clothes, smacking their lips, or saying something confused or inappropriate. These actions are called automisms and a person has no memory of them or of any other event that takes place during his or her seizure. Occasionally more complicated automisms occur; for example, a person having a seizure in a shop might walk away with an item unpaid for. This sort of automism can easily be misunderstood and lead to distressing consequences. All these kinds of complex partial seizure are usually followed by a period during which the person appears confused, not knowing where he or she is or should be doing, before he or she returns completely to normal.

It is thought that complex partial seizures arise because of the spread of abnormal electrical activity from either the frontal or most commonly temporal lobe into the closely related limbic system. The limbic system consists of a number of structures deep within the temporal lobe and frontal lobe of the brain that deal with primitive aspects of memory, behaviour and bodily function, so that many temporal lobe partial seizures that begin with simple symptoms can become complex during the course of the seizure. Alternatively, if the seizure begins in or very close to the limbic system, particularly in the frontal lobe, the person might lose awareness from the start. As we shall see, this kind of seizure can look like petit mal *(see page 19)*. But it is quite different. It is a partial

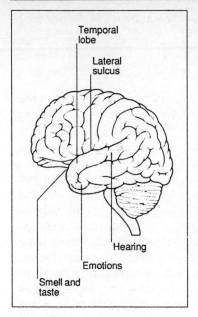

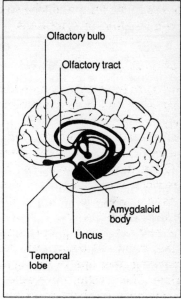

The temporal lobe and some of its functions.

The relationship between the temporal lobe and the limbic system deep inside the brain.

rather than a generalized seizure and needs different treatment.

Partial seizures that become generalized

One characteristic of the electrical discharge at the basis of seizures is its tendency to spread from the site of onset to other parts of the brain. As we have seen, simple partial seizures can spread to other parts of the hemisphere from where they start. They can also spread to the other hemisphere, resulting in a generalized seizure, which almost always takes the tonic-clonic form. An attack of this kind, that results from spread, is usually recognizable because of the particular preliminary symptoms.

Generalized seizures

A generalized seizure is one in which the disturbed electrical activity of the seizure affects the whole of both hemispheres of the brain. It is likely that disturbed activity in the deep structure of the brain is involved in this kind of seizure.

Tonic-clonic (grand mal) seizures

This common type of seizure can arise either because of the spread of seizure activity following a partial seizure or directly, when it is called a primary generalized seizure. In the former the person suffering the seizure will have symptoms of a partial seizure (an aura), followed by a typical tonic-clonic seizure. In tonic-clonic seizures that are generalized from the start the person does not experience an aura, but loses consciousness immediately.

During the initial tonic phase of the fit all the muscles of the body contract and the person becomes rigid. If his bladder is full, the contraction of the muscles there will result in urination. As the muscles in the lungs contract, they force air out through the vocal cords and the person seems to cry out. Breathing might stop for a short while and the person become rather blue as a result. This tonic phase usually lasts for less than a minute, although it might well seem considerably longer, and is followed by the clonic, or jerking, phase. Jerking is caused by phases of relaxation alternating with further muscular contractions. During this part of the fit a person might bite his or her tongue.

After a minute or two of a clonic phase, the fit ends and the person relaxes. He or she will then be deeply unconscious and unrousable. Consciousness returns gradually and within five minutes the individual might be talking, although he will appear rather confused or irritable. He will want simply to be left alone and might become a little aggressive if interfered with. As consciousness improves, the person will begin to behave more normally, but he might have no memory for 45 minutes to an hour after the fit. Very often a person remains sleepy and has an unpleasant headache for some time.

There are several other, rarer, types of generalized seizure. They all tend to show themselves first in children and none of

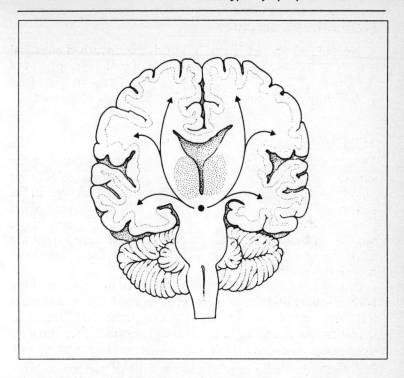

A seizure which is generalized from the onset. The person will not experience an aura.

them arises because of spread after a partial fit. Let us consider these in a little more detail.

Simple absence (petit mal)

This type of seizure is characterized by a sudden, usually momentary absence during which a child loses contact with his or her surroundings, stops whatever he is doing, and might flutter his eyelids. Very often these attacks are so short that they are not recognized by school friends, parents or teachers, and the child who has them is often unaware that they are happening. They can occur many times a day, and sometimes they are so frequent that they interfere with a child's concentration and performance at school.

Everyone is familiar with the term 'petit mal', but it is often wrongly used to describe any kind of minor epileptic attack. We should avoid this. Simple absences are an unusual and very specific kind of seizure. They should not be confused with other trance-like seizures, such as the more common complex partial seizures, which demand quite different treatment.

Myoclonic jerks

Myoclonus is a sudden, brief, involuntary jerk, which can affect the whole body, but usually involves the arms, upper body and sometimes the head. These seizures happen most often in the morning within an hour or so of waking. They are not usually associated with any alteration in consciousness, although sometimes they are accompanied by a brief absence similar to petit mal.

Complex absences

These are seizures that children who often have some underlying brain damage have and they can recur frequently. The absences are longer than simple absences and much more often associated with either massive jerks or sudden loss of muscle power (atonic attacks), both of which can cause the children to be thrown off their feet. Because of the very sudden onset of the attack and lack of warning, children may injure themselves. Many children suffering this unpleasant kind of attack need to wear protective helmets to avoid head injuries.

When do seizures take place?

Although for a lot of people seizures happen unpredictably, for others patterns of attacks can be identified. Sometimes knowing about these patterns may help precipitating factors to be avoided, so that the frequency of attacks may be reduced.

The sleep-waking cycle

It is not unusual for people to have seizures only while they are asleep. When tonic-clonic seizures happen at this time, they usually have a localized onset; indeed, an EEG recording *(see page 48)* during sleep is often used to test people who have partial seizures for localized abnormalities.

Some people have generalized seizures, such as myoclonus, absence or tonic-clonic seizures, within an hour or two of waking. They often find that missing sleep is a powerful provocative factor. Attacks tend to take place after a late night, particularly if the person has been drinking alcohol *(see page 96)*.

During the day fits are more likely to occur when people are bored or apathetic. This should always be borne in mind. Although an active sport such as football might be thought of as slightly risky for a boy with epilepsy, he is more likely to have a seizure if he is sitting indoors by himself while his friends are out playing than if he is out on the football field enjoying himself.

The reproductive cycle

Very often women with epilepsy have seizures related to their menstrual cycle. They usually happen a few days before or just after the beginning of a period. We are not certain why this is. One possibility is that there are changes in the fluid balance of the body and the brain that make seizures more likely during this time. It is also possible that changes in hormonal balance are involved. In spite of this, the oral contraceptive pill seems safe for women with epilepsy and hardly ever has any effect on the occurrence of seizures *(see page 81)*. Taking the drug clobazam in addition to your usual drugs for about five days before and after the first day of a period can sometimes help *(see page 112)*.

Stress factors

Many people with epilepsy say that their seizures are more frequent and troublesome when they are emotionally distressed or upset. There is certainly an important link between the way people feel and their likelihood of having an attack. Sleep is often disturbed by anxiety or depression, and people may be less consistent about taking their anti-epileptic medication when they are depressed. It must be emphasized that although psychological factors can make seizures more likely if you have epilepsy, they cannot by themselves cause epilepsy, which is a physical disorder.

First Aid during and after fits

Do

- Try to move away any objects that might be a danger to the person having the attack. If this is impossible, and only then, you should consider moving the person.

- Try to lay the person down comfortably, usually on the floor or ground, and loosen any tight clothing.

- Try to settle the person comfortably in a semi-prone position on the floor or ground as soon as he or she is relaxed after the end of a fit. Then leave him or her to come round slowly. If you interfere with a person during this phase, you might be pushed away or lashed out at in confusion.

- Call an ambulance or a doctor immediately only if someone is having a succession of fits without regaining consciousness between them, which indicates status epilepticus *(see page 129)*.

Don't

- Interfere with a person unnecessarily during a tonic or clonic phase of a seizure. In particular, don't try to introduce spoons or fingers into his mouth in an attempt to prevent him biting his tongue. More damage is usually done by spoons or other implements than by the fit itself.

- Call an ambulance or doctor if someone is having a simple, uncomplicated fit.

Reflex seizures

Some people have fits in particular circumstances. Probably

the most common of this type of seizure are febrile convulsions. These happen to children up to the age of five only when they have a high temperature *(see pages 36–9)*. Other people are sensitive to flashing lights, which are used as a test to provoke seizures during standard EEG examinations. The usual sources of flashing lights are discotheques and faulty cathode ray tubes in televisions. The flickering television image is particularly powerful in causing seizures. Nevertheless, this kind of trigger is unusual, and working with computers and visual display units (VDUS) is almost always safe. Only 3–5 per cent of people with epilepsy have seizures provoked in this way.

Now that we have described the common kinds of epileptic seizure, we need to look at the different types of epilepsy – the pattern of recurrent seizures.

3

Types of epilepsy

People with epilepsy can suffer more than one type of seizure and we identify epileptic disorders by the following information:

- the kinds of seizures that occur
- the age at which the seizures started
- whether the epilepsy is likely to be inherited
- the degree to which the cause is identifiable

It is important to recognize the different patterns of epilepsy because:

- the type of special investigations needed can be different
- the treatment can be different
- the outlook for the control of the condition can vary considerably

The table opposite is a simplified list of the different types of epilepsy. Let's look first at the generalized epilepsies with seizures that are generalized from the onset. We can subdivide these into:

- idiopathic epilepsies, which are usually inherited
- symptomatic epilepsies, which are the result of identified brain damage or disease

Cryptogenic is a term which indicates that while we think the epilepsy has a cause, we can't identify what it is.

Idiopathic Generalized Epilepsies

These are epilepsies with no identifiable cause. People with them have no obvious brain damage or disease and their brains are normal apart from their susceptibility to seizures. It is quite common to find a family history of this form of epilepsy and it certainly has a genetic basis, that is, it can be inherited. These kinds of epilepsy very rarely start before the age of three or after the age of 30 and the EEGs of people with them show a generalized spike-and-wave disturbance.

Classification of the epilepsies

Generalized epilepsies

Idiopathic
   Childhood absence
   Juvenile Myoclonic Epilepsy
   Tonic-clonic awakening epilepsy

Usually symptomatic
   Infantile spasm syndrome
   Lennox-Gastaut syndrome
   Early myoclonic epilepsies

Partial epilepsies

Idiopathic
   Benign focal motor epilepsy of childhood
   Benign occipital epilepsy of childhood

Usually symptomatic
   Simple partial epilepsies
   Complex partial epilepsies

Specific epileptic syndromes

Febrile convulsions

Reflex epilepsies

Stress-induced seizures

Unclassified epilepsies

Neonatal seizures

Nocturnal tonic-clonic seizures (normal EEGs)

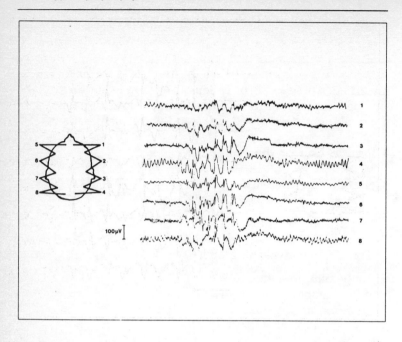

A burst of generalized spike wave discharge in the eeg affecting both sides of the brain simultaneously.

Childhood and juvenile absence (petit mal) epilepsy

Childhood absence epilepsy is a rare disorder and affects only about 3 per cent of people with epilepsy. Forty per cent of children with this epilepsy have relatives with the condition. They have typical absence seizures *(see page 19)*, which usually begin between the ages of five and ten, and rarely, if ever, continue in adult life, although around one third of them may have occasional tonic-clonic waking seizures in later life. The disorder shows a very specific EEG abnormality and is characterized by a three-cycles-per-second spike-and-wave EEG pattern *(see figure)*. It responds well to drug treatment and in the majority of cases people can discontinue therapy in adulthood. Jane's case is a good example.

Jane was seven years old when her parents began to notice that she would stop what she was doing for a second or two,

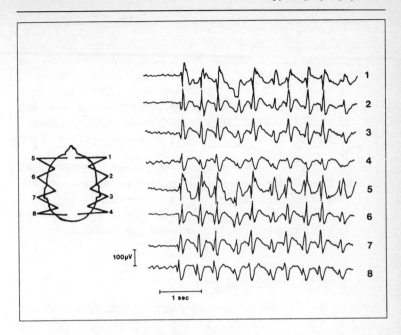

The eeg during a petit mal absence showing synchronous regular spike wave activity at three cycles per second on both sides of the brain.

or not reply to a question. They thought that she was daydreaming and were not worried. At first this happened infrequently, but by the time Jane was nine her teachers were concerned about her progress at school and complained about her poor concentration. One morning while Jane was getting ready for school her mother heard her give a brief cry, followed by the sound of her falling. She ran to the bedroom to find Jane having a convulsion.

The family doctor referred Jane to a paediatric specialist at the local hospital and an EEG was arranged. It showed that she was having brief absences associated with bursts of three-cycles-per-second spike-and-wave discharges. There was no doubt that Jane's daydreaming and poor concentration were due to petit mal epilepsy.

Jane was started on treatment with a small dose of sodium valproate. Her parents and teachers were now looking out for Jane's absences, and noticed that they were very greatly reduced. After six months the absences appeared to have stopped. Jane remained very well and a repeat EEG taken when she was 12 was normal. It was decided to withdraw her medication gradually.

Jane's absences did not return and she suffered only two further seizures: a tonic-clonic seizure early one morning when she was 19 and had been out late at a party the previous evening, and another one when she was 23, six weeks after the birth of her first child.

In some people absences may begin after puberty. When they do, they are less frequent, but more often associated with myoclonic jerks and tonic-clonic seizures than when they begin in childhood. This is called juvenile absence epilepsy and it is less likely to disappear in adult life than is childhood absence.

Juvenile Myoclonic epilepsy

This epilepsy is characterized by early morning myoclonic jerks *(see page 20)* that affect mainly the arms. Although it is not usually associated with absence, some people do experience brief absence. On some mornings myoclonic jerking might be very frequent and develop into a tonic-clonic fit. The response to treatment is excellent, but prolonged therapy is often necessary, as withdrawal of the drugs can lead to a recurrence of seizures. This is what happened in John's case.

John's father had been discharged from the army because he had had two tonic-clonic seizures at the age of 20. He had been treated for a brief period with phenobarbitone and had remained well. John was 17 when he began to experience jerks of his arms soon after getting up in the morning. At first John and his parents assumed this was nothing more than clumsiness and as he always seemed to improve by the time he had to go to work, they did nothing about it.

John noticed that the jerks seemed to be more of a problem if he had been up late the night before. One Saturday morning after a night out drinking with his friends his jerks were particularly severe and he decided to go back to bed. Half an hour later his father found John in a confused state, having bitten his tongue and wet the bed.

John's doctor sent him to the hospital for investigation. The neurologist there arranged an EEG. Bursts of generalized spike-and-wave activity showed up and when John was tested by being exposed to a flashing light these became more marked. The neurologist told John and his parents that he had a form of myoclonic epilepsy and started his treatment with sodium valproate *(see page 115)*. John was told that he would have to give up his provisional driving licence for the present.

To start with, John's morning jerks became far less frequent, but his medication had to be increased before they stopped completely. After two years without a fit John was eager to try to do without his medication, but, unfortunately, soon after reducing the dose he again had morning jerks. John decided to stay on his previous dosage to ensure that he had no further fits and would be eligible for a driving licence.

Wakening tonic-clonic epilepsy

Tonic-clonic seizures can begin in childhood or adolescence. There is no specific aura to the attacks, and they tend to be infrequent and to happen shortly after waking. Treatment for this epilepsy is very effective. It usually ceases soon after medication is started and people may no longer need treatment after fits have been controlled for two to three years. Even if they start again, attacks tend to get less frequent as people get older.

Symptomatic generalized epilpsies

Children who have suffered some brain damage very early in their lives may have these disorders. They are characterized by many different kinds of seizures, including complex absence seizures, often associated with myoclonus and atonic attacks, and frequent tonic-clonic seizures.

Infantile spasms

This is the most severe and difficult epilepsy occurring in childhood. Attacks usually begin between four and seven months of age, and rarely after 12 months. The most frequent attacks are what are called salaam spasms, when the child's head suddenly and forcefully bends forward while the knees bend and arms flex. Most infants with this epilepsy are brain damaged before they develop these fits, most often by a condition called tuberose sclerosis, but a few children's retardation is noticed only after the fits have begun. Later the child may have seizures characteristic of the Lennox-Gastaut Syndrome (see below) or a variety of partial seizures.

The condition is associated with a very striking EEG abnormality called hypsarrythmia which affects all the brain. This led to the condition being thought of as a generalized epilepsy, but new information makes this doubtful. PET scanning studies have suggested the epilepsy may arise in one, not both, hemispheres and vigabatrin, a new drug for partial epilepsies, seems very effective in many children.

In the past treatment was usually with adrenocorticotrophic hormone (ACTH), but children with this condition often did poorly, both in terms of controlling the epilepsy and in terms of their development. Vigabatrin, at least in the short term, may suppress seizures satisfactorily, but we don't yet know how it might affect development in the longer term.

The Lennox-Gastaut syndrome

This begins slightly later than infantile spasms – most often between the ages of one and three years, and rarely up to the age of seven or eight. It might account for up to 10 per cent of all epilepsies and is approximately twice as common as childhood absence epilepsy.

Children with the Lennox-Gastaut Syndrome have frequent seizures of different kinds. Usually they have typical absence seizures (see page 19), which are often associated with myoclonic jerks, tonic seizures (when the body goes into a spasm), or atonic drop attacks (when the body suddenly loses all its muscular support). They may also have more typical tonic-clonic attacks.

The attacks tend to be difficult to control and absence status is common. This is a state in which children have a series of absences over a long period, which makes them behave in a confused way. The condition can be very difficult to diagnose unless an EEG is done. There is often mental retardation from an early age and it can become worse because of the child's epilepsy. Seizures usually continue into adult life, but can

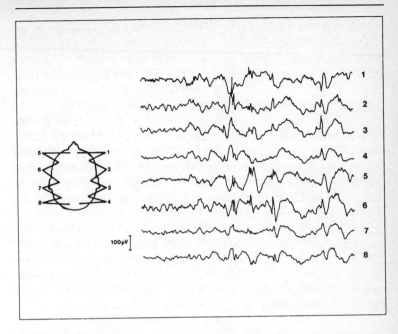

Generalized irregular spike wave activity. This person had symptomatic generalized epilepsy.

sometimes change to become more typical complex partial seizures. Michael's case is typical.

Michael was his mother's first child. She had been in labour for six hours when the midwives became concerned that the baby's heart rate was increasing in an irregular way. Because of this, Michael was delivered by forceps and it was clear that he was far from well. He was taken to the hospital's special baby care unit and placed on a ventilator for four days because he was not breathing very well. During this time he had brief seizures and was given drugs to suppress them as well as calcium to correct a low level in his blood. Michael gradually improved and left the hospital two months later.

Michael did not have any further treatment until he was two years old. However, during this time his parents noticed that he was not developing as quickly as they expected. By the time he was two and a half he had not begun to walk and had been crawling for only three months. His parents became concerned when Michael began to have brief episodes in which he would suddenly jump as though he had been startled, very often falling over. Then he caught a cold and became feverish. His mother found him having a convulsion in his cot and took him to the hospital.

The paediatricians believed Michael had developed a form of epilepsy that was probably caused by brain damage that had occurred around the time of his birth. He was started on drug treatment. Unfortunately, although many different drugs were tried, none controlled his fits satisfactorily. He had attacks on most days and they could occur several times a day. They mostly took the form of brief muscle jerks that would often throw him off his feet. Michael would hurt himself during the attacks, so Michael's doctor arranged for him to wear a special head protector. Less frequently, he had attacks when his body suddenly became stiff and rigid for 10 to 15 seconds. Every two to three weeks he had a tonic-clonic seizure and after these his parents noticed that his other, more minor seizures were less frequent.

As the years went by Michael's disabilities became more obvious and it was clear that he could not be properly cared for at his local school. He went to a special school, but he never learned to read and write satisfactorily, and he remained very dependent on his parents. By the age of 15 his attacks had begun to change. He had fewer of the myoclonic attacks and began to have episodes when he would go into a trance-like state and pick at his clothes in an abstracted and fidgety way. His drugs were changed, but while a combination of phenytoin, valproate and carbamazepine reduced the number of tonic-clonic seizures he was having to six or seven a year, the new complex partial seizures were still frequent.

A few times Michael became very unsteady and sleepy after an increase in the dose of his phenytoin and the doctors realized he was reacting to the drugs. From then on he had to have regular blood tests to prevent the chances of further drug intoxication.

Michael continued to suffer from severe epilepsy throughout his life. At the age of 20 he was admitted to one of the special centres for epilepsy for a period of assessment and rehabilitation. After this he was able to undertake some light work, which he thoroughly enjoyed.

Partial epilepsies

These make up about 60 per cent of all epilepsies. People with these kinds of epilepsy have partial seizures with or without tonic-clonic attacks. They can develop in childhood, or commonly begin at a later age; virtually everyone developing epilepsy after the age of 30 has a partial epilepsy, even those who appear to have only tonic-clonic attacks. Often their grand mal attacks happen when they are asleep and therefore unaware of an aura, which would indicate the localized origin.

Doctors can identify a particular cause for a partial epilepsy more often than they can for a generalized one. It can develop after severe head injuries and strokes, and very occasionally is due to a brain abscess or tumour. It can occur following damage to the brain during severe febrile seizures or because of structural abnormalities of the brain's development. None the less, in many cases no cause for a partial epilepsy can be found.

Benign (Rolandic) focal motor epilepsy of childhood

This is an idiopathic probably genetic epilepsy in which children between the ages of eight and 12 years begin to have simple motor seizures *(see page 11)*. These are often relatively few and disappear as the child grows up. Tonic-clonic seizures are rare. Some paediatricians think very mild forms of this kind of epilepsy are so benign that they may not be worth treating. That is what was decided in Mary's case.

Mary woke one night when she was 11 years old because her right hand was jerking. She became frightened when she found she couldn't stop it and called out to her mother. Almost as soon as her mother arrived in the bedroom the jerking stopped. During the next year a similar sequence of events happened three times and Mary's parents took her to see their doctor, who sent her to a specialist. Mary's EEG was abnormal with some spikes that were localized over the central region of the left side of the head.

The specialist reassured Mary and her parents that she had a very mild epileptic condition, and emphasized that these kind of attacks continued for a brief period of a person's life and only during sleep. In view of the infrequency of Mary's attacks, he thought that it was not necessary to treat her with anti-epileptic drugs. Mary's parents agreed when it was explained that taking drugs might have some minor effects on Mary's concentration and memory. Mary continued to have occasional attacks until she was 14, when they stopped.

More rarely, children can have a similar benign epilepsy with seizures arising in the occipital lobe and causing visual disturbance *(see page 15)*.

Autosomal dominant nocturnal frontal lobe epilepsy

This is a very rare condition but is important and interesting because it is the first human epilepsy to have its genetic basis identified. It is due to an error in the genetic material (DNA) which codes for a part of the neurone membrane that recognizes a neurotransmitter called acetylcholine. In the coming years many more such epilepsies with different errors in coding will be discovered.

Symptomatic partial epilepsy

These epilepsies are caused by damage to different lobes of the brain, most commonly the temporal (70 per cent of cases) or frontal lobes (20 per cent of cases), by many different conditions *(see above)*.

Temporal lobe epilepsy

People with this condition most commonly have complex partial seizures *(see page 16)*. They might first experience an aura, suggesting an origin in the temporal lobe, followed by a trance-like state and automatism. They might also have tonic-clonic seizures. This kind of epilepsy is important for three reasons:

1. It is very common.
2. Because it is difficult to control completely, it tends to cause more problems both to people with the condition and their doctors than most other epilepsies. While drug treatment will usually prevent the tonic-clonic seizures, it is often

difficult to abolish the trance-like attacks, and about 50 per cent of people with it continue to have attacks and remain in long-term treatment.

3. People who have this kind of epilepsy are more likely than other people to suffer from nervous and psychiatric disorders. Fortunately, these disorders are usually quite mild, but they can include anxiety, depression and personality problems.

Although there is no simple and certain explanation for the connection between this kind of epilepsy and psychiatric disorders, there are some possibilities:

1. Because temporal lobe epilepsy is difficult to control, people who have it tend to have more disturbance in their lives, and depression could be a natural reaction to this.
2. Some anti-epileptic drugs seem to contribute to psychiatric symptoms and people with this epilepsy are often placed on larger doses of more drugs than others.
3. As the temporal lobe is important to emotions and other sensations, it is possible that disturbance in this part of the brain is responsible for both the epilepsy and psychiatric problems.

Medial temporal epilepsy

This particular kind of temporal lobe epilepsy is common and very important because it is often treated successfully with surgery. People with this epilepsy often have convulsions, with fever, in childhood, but the attacks are longer than the typical febrile seizures that are so common. After one or two convulsions like this, there are often no more problems until later childhood, when typical complex partial seizures begin, usually preceded by an aura that may include a feeling in the stomach, a smell, a taste in the mouth or *déjà vu*. Tonic-clonic seizures occur rarely once treatment is started and usually during sleep. Modern magnetic resonance (MR) scanning shows scarring of the hippocampus of the temporal lobe, usually just on one side. If this is removed, 70–80 per cent of people who would otherwise be very disabled by their epilepsy can be cured.

Which are the commonest types of epilepsy?

We have already shown how common the condition itself is *(see page 1)*, but it may be interesting to know how many people get which type of seizure. The table below shows the results of a study done in Denmark in 1983. Clearly the tonic-clonic seizures make up the largest proportion.

Special situation epilepsies

Febrile convulsions

These happen most commonly to children between the ages of nine and 20 months. The convulsions do not seem to take place before six months or after five years of age. The condition is completely different from other infantile and childhood epilepsies, as seizures take place only when children have a temperature higher than 100.4°F (38° C); the normal body temperature is 98.6° F (37° C).

Incidence of Seizure Types

	Per cent
Primary tonic-clonic	25.6
Petit mal	3.9
Myoclonic seizures	3.1
Simple partial seizures	4.9
Complex partial seizures	17.9
Partial and tonic-clonic	14.4
Alcohol-induced seizures	6.3
Stress-induced seizures	8.0
Drug-induced seizures	1.3
Isolated unprovoked seizures	13.4
Unclassified	1.2
Total	100

About 5 per cent of children have febrile convulsions. The susceptibility runs in families and up to 30 per cent of children suffering febrile convulsions have a near relative who also had them. The attacks usually take the form of tonic-clonic seizures and happen as a fever reaches its peak. Sometimes a convulsion is the first symptom that a child is developing a feverish illness. The convulsions occur usually with simple virus infections, such as coughs and colds, but also with measles and mumps and more serious illnesses, such as pneumonia, gastroenteritis and, occasionally, meningitis. Usually a convulsion takes place only once. Sometimes, though, there is a repeat, particularly if:

- the first convulsion happened before the age of one year
- the child has had previous brain damage
- other members of the family have had the same condition

The chance of children who have febrile convulsions having epilepsy later in life is very low, perhaps as little as 5 per cent. David's case was one of these.

When David was two years old he developed a high fever during a bout of tonsillitis. His mother found him stiff, blue and convulsing. She called the family doctor, who came to the house within 20 minutes. David was still convulsing and the doctor immediately called an ambulance to take him to the local hospital. He was given emergency treatment, which stopped his convulsion, but by that time he probably had been fitting for over an hour. David quickly recovered from this illness and had no further problems until he was 10.

Then David's parents began to notice that he would sometimes stare to one side and swallow. This did not happen often, but when it did, it seemed to upset David. By the time he was 15 he could describe some of the feelings he experienced at these times: he had a peculiar taste in his mouth, followed quickly by a frightening sensation he couldn't describe. When he was 16, his parents found him having a tonic-clonic seizure in his sleep one night.

David was sent to the hospital, where an EEG showed an abnormality in the right temporal lobe. He was told that his attacks were those of a temporal lobe epilepsy, probably caused by damage from his prolonged febrile convulsion. At first he was given phenytoin and the prescription was later changed to carbamazepine. The drugs reduced the frequency of his attacks to once or twice a month and stopped the tonic-clonic seizures.

David completed his school career successfully, doing well in his examinations, and when went on to work for his father as a salesman. But his attacks became longer lasting and more embarrassing. During an attack he would walk about in a confused way, often spitting on the floor. This was followed by quite long periods of confusion, and so it became more and more difficult for him to do his job satisfactorily.

When he was 20 his specialist decided that David should have further, more complex investigations so that the site of onset of his seizures could be discovered. The tests showed that his seizures originated in the right anterior temporal lobe, and it was felt that this could be removed without causing David any harm. After the operation, David had only one more seizure, after three months, and years later is taking only a small dose of carbamazepine.

Treatment of febrile convulsions

The first step is to stop the seizure itself. In most cases febrile seizures stop of their own accord after a short period. If a child continues to convulse for more than five to ten minutes, you must call a doctor or take the child to the nearest hospital casualty department as quickly as possible. This is important because very rarely febrile seizures cause brain damage; a high fever seems to increase the possibility of damage to the brain cells during convulsions. The child should probably be taken to the hospital in any case, so that the cause of the fever can be discovered and any possible infection treated.

Should children who have had an episode of febrile convulsions be treated with anti-epileptic drugs? Although there is some evidence that taking drugs such as phenobarbitone and sodium valproate may reduce the risk of further seizures, this seems unnecessary for most children who have had only a single convulsion. All that is needed is for the parents to watch any feverish illness very carefully. You should treat rising temperature by removing the bedclothes and sponging your child with tepid water to keep the body temperature down. Some doctors might also suggest your giving the drug diazepam rectally if a seizure takes place.

Anti-epileptic drugs may be necessary for children who are at particular high risk of further attacks. These are children:

- whose first convulsion happened before the age of one year
- who have shown signs of brain damage
- who have a strong family history of febrile convulsions
- whose first febrile convulsion was particularly long or confined to one side of the body

Reflex epilepsies

Some people have epileptic attacks brought on by particular circumstances, such as flashing lights. A sensitivity to flashing lights is not common. Only 2 to 3 per cent of people with epilepsy have it, but people suspected of being epileptic are usually exposed to flashing lights in their EEG investigations. Susceptible people show an abnormal EEG pattern. As soon as this appears, the EEG technician can turn off the lights and the person will not realize that anything unusual has happened. However, if a susceptible person is exposed to a flashing light for a longer period, he or she may have a seizure. This is most likely to happen when the person tries to adjust a flickering television set. It can happen when you are driving along a sunlit road with regularly spaced trees, causing dazzling flashes. Flashing lights at a discotheque rarely provoke this kind of attack.

There has been more concern recently about this kind of epilepsy as children spend more time watching television or playing computer games. If a child is unfortunate enough to have photosensitive epilepsy, a number of simple precautions reduce the risk of seizures:

- Keep as far away from the screen as possible and use a remote control to change channels and adjust the set. The less of the field of vision the television takes up, the less the risk.
- Always watch the screen in a well lit room, never in the dark where the television is the only source of light.

Other, much rarer reflex epilepsies are caused by particular sounds or music, or even complicated tasks such as mental arithmetic.

4

Diagnosing epilepsy

We have seen that there are many types of epileptic seizures, with extremely varied effects, and they can produce unusual and strange sensations. How, then, can your doctor be certain that you have epilepsy? The diagnosis can be very simple and straightforward if you have an aura that is easy to describe, and if your attacks have been witnessed by another person who can describe them to the doctor. An accurate eyewitness account of what happened during an attack is the most useful factor in deciding whether or not you have epilepsy. So it is important for you to try to take an eyewitness with you when you visit the doctor who is investigating any possible epilepsy. You should also be prepared for the doctor's questions and the checklist on page 42 will be helpful.

Without these clues the diagnosis of epilepsy can be difficult. If you do not have an aura, or have one that is very difficult to describe, and there are no eyewitnesses to your attacks, it might be impossible to reach a firm diagnosis using your account alone. Then investigations may be helpful in coming to a decision. It is best both for you and your doctor to keep an open mind about the nature of your attacks rather than immediately presume they are epileptic. A lot of people have been wrongly diagnosed as having epilepsy – up to 20 per cent of people admitted to special epilepsy centres turn out not to have it and yet may have had years of inappropriate treatment. The diagnosis of epilepsy has such important implications for the person involved and his or her family that everyone developing symptoms should see a neurologist, paediatrician or other doctor specializing in epilepsy.

Confusion with non-epileptic attacks

It is important to distinguish between epileptic attacks and other causes of loss or alteration of consciousness.

Checklist: What the doctor wants to know

1. Was there a warning immediately before the attack?

2. Can you describe this warning easily and clearly?

3. Is there an eyewitness who can talk to the doctor?

4. What happened during the attack?

5. How long did the attack last?

6. How did you feel and behave after the attack?

7. Have you had just one kind of attack or more than one?

8. Have you had any other recent illnesses or symptoms?

9. At the time of the attack had you had any alcohol or taken any drugs?

10. Does anyone else in your family have epilepsy or blackouts?

11. If you have consulted other doctors:

    • who were they?
    • when did you see them?
    • where did you see them?
    • what investigations did you have?
    • what treatment did they advise?

Stroke

Sometimes people are unclear as to the difference between a seizure and a stroke. A stroke is due to a disturbance of blood supply to the brain and results in an area of brain damage. Its symptoms can come on quickly, but recovery is very slow, usually taking weeks. It is usually older people who have strokes, whereas epileptic seizures are more common among younger ones.

Fainting

Many people have fainted at some time in their lives. It is a normal phenomenon caused by your blood pressure falling to such a low level that it is insufficient to pump blood from your heart up to your head. If your brain does not get enough blood which carries oxygen, you begin to feel lightheaded and quickly become pale, sweaty and slightly nauseated. You may begin to feel that the world is rotating around you and your vision might become dim, losing the normal appreciation of colour. You will know that you are going to 'black out' and you may feel that you are detached or drifting away.

These feelings are most severe when you are standing up and are a clear indication that you should lie down. Lying down or putting your head between your knees usually will make you feel better immediately. Too often, however, people feel they need fresh air and try to walk to an exit, and then they are likely to lose consciousness.

When you faint, you fall to the ground gracefully and rarely injure yourself. Your body is floppy and motionless while you remain unconscious, although some people's bodies jerk a few times, sometimes quite dramatically. As soon as you have fallen, your head is on a level with your heart, so circulation to the brain returns and you start to regain consciousness almost immediately. Because of this, in the majority of cases there is no confusion between fainting and epilepsy.

Unfortunately, some people are unaware that the act of fainting itself soon restores consciousness and they will try to help someone who has fainted by picking him or her up. Doing this can prolong the period during which the blood is not reaching the brain and might even cause the person to have a typical tonic-clonic seizure. This is not an epileptic seizure and a diagnosis of epilepsy should not be accepted if there is a history of faintness before a seizure.

The differences between fainting and epileptic seizures are listed on page 44. One of the most useful clues is the circumstances in which fainting tends to occur. It is most likely to happen when you are standing still, usually in hot, crowded places such as bars, discotheques and underground trains. Unpleasant circumstances, such as the sight of blood or an accident, or having an injection, can also cause fainting. In summary, it is usually provoked, unlike seizures, which are unpredictable.

Fainting is most common among teenagers and young adults, and is more frequent among women – particularly around the time of their periods – than men. When the cause of fainting is obvious, you do not need to have tests or investigations. However, old people may faint due to dehydration or heart problems, so it is wise to consult a doctor if an old person has fainted. He or she should be investigated and treated appropriately.

Factors differentiating faints and fits

	Faints	Fits
Posture	Upright	Any posture
Pallor and sweating	Invariable	Uncommon
Onset	Gradual	Sudden/Aura
Injury	Rare	Can occur
Convulsive jerks	Sometimes	Common
Incontinence	Rare	Common
Unconsciousness	Seconds	Minutes
Recovery	Rapid	Often slow
Following confusion	Rare	Common
Frequency	Infrequent	Can be frequent
Precipitating factors	Crowded places Lack of food Unpleasant circumstances	Rare

Hyperventilation attacks

If you have ever had to blow up an airbed without a pump, you will know that taking very deep breaths over a long time can make you feel peculiar. Many people who are anxious tend to overbreathe slightly. When they become particularly panicky, the overbreathing can increase and cause a variety of symptoms that might be wrongly attributed to an epileptic seizure, including:

- tingling and spasms of the hands
- nausea
- lightheadedness and even some alteration of consciousness

This is because overbreathing blows off a gas, carbon dioxide, from the blood. Carbon dioxide concentration in the blood is important in controlling circulation to the brain. Very low concentrations of carbon dioxide cause the blood vessels to constrict and reduce the supply of blood to the head and extremities, producing these symptoms.

Rage outbursts

Although it is true that some people with temporal lobe epilepsy experience altered emotions and become confused, violent behaviour during attacks is exceedingly rare. In spite of this, epilepsy is sometimes suggested as the cause when people with short tempers lose control of themselves. Such outbursts of rage are usually provoked, no matter how trivial the cause, and are rarely stereotyped in the way epileptic seizures are. There must be exceptionally firm evidence of an epileptic basis for such outbursts before they are treated as being epileptic.

Pseudoseizures

These are attacks that are feigned, either consciously or subconsciously. They are often used as a means of manipulating people, including the person's family and doctor. For this reason pseudoseizures almost always occur in someone else's presence and they tend to be very dramatic. They are usually less stereotyped than epileptic attacks and often more violent, the arms and legs thrashing about in a very wild manner. They can be particularly difficult to deal with, especially when someone with genuine epilepsy also has pseudoseizures. This is not uncommon, and making the distinction between true seizures and pseudoseizures may mean that intensive investigation is necessary.

What are the causes of epilepsy?

Deciding that someone has epileptic seizures is not itself a complete diagnosis because seizures can happen for many reasons. For example, we know that someone who has meningitis may have a seizure. This is not epilepsy; the underlying illness is the cause of the attacks and successful treatment will also cure the attacks. Chronic epilepsy can be brought on by a number of conditions affecting the brain, some of which are associated with specific age groups. At present we cannot detect a definite cause for epilepsy in about 50 per cent of cases, but this figure is falling as our investigations improve.

Brain disorders causing seizures and epilepsy

Idiopathic	Inherited genetic epilepsies
Congenital	Birth trauma, tuberose sclerosis, arterio-venous malformation
Infections	Meningitis, encephalitis, abscess
Trauma	Severe concussion, haematoma (extradural, subdural, intracerebral), depressed fracture
Tumour	
Stroke	

Neonatal epilepsy

In newborn babies seizures are most likely to develop if:

- there was a problem with the delivery
- the baby has been starved of oxygen
- the baby has low blood sugar or low blood calcium

Seizures that begin after the first week and during the first year of life often reflect brain damage that occurred before or during birth. Epilepsies in the first year of life starting after the immediate time of birth tend to be relatively severe and difficult to control *(see Infantile Spasms, page 29; Lennox-Gastaut Syndrome, page 30)*.

Childhood epilepsies

Epilepsy beginning in a toddler is most likely to be a form of generalized epilepsy *(see pages 24–25)*. It can be constitutional and, occasionally, inherited. Infections of the brain are a significant cause for epilepsy at this age, as in brain damage *(see Lennox-Gastaut Syndrome, page 30)*. Epilepsy in a toddler must be distinguished from febrile convulsions *(see page 36)*.

Teenage and adult epilepsies

Juvenile myoclonic and absence epilepsies can begin during the teenage years, but not often after the age of 20 or 25. After this, partial epilepsies, which can begin at any age, are the most common type of epilepsy. A person developing partial epilepsy between the ages of 25 and 60 may need investigations to exclude the remote possibility of a brain tumour.

Excessive drinking and head injury are common causes of epilepsy at this age, although head injury is an overestimated cause. Probably everyone bangs his head at some time, but epilepsy can be attributed to an incident of that sort only if there was a severe injury with prolonged unconsciousness or confusion, or a depressed skull fracture.

Epilepsy and old age

Narrowing of the blood vessels is probably the commonest cause of old people developing epilepsy. Some people develop it as a result of strokes caused by narrowing of blood vessels to the brain. Others have transient ischaemic attacks (TIAS). These are minor strokes that produce short-lasting symptoms and they need to be distinguished from epileptic seizures.

Distinguishing fits from TIAS is usually very straightforward. TIAS don't generally cause loss of consciousness and they are almost always longer lasting than fits would be. However, if you think an elderly relative is experiencing either fits or TIAS you should ask your doctor. He or she is the person who must differentiate between these two.

People who develop epilepsy in old age have partial seizures, often going on to tonic-clonic seizures during sleep. They can usually be treated successfully with drugs and epilepsy in old age is rarely a major problem.

In the next pages we explain how doctors diagnose the different forms of epilepsy, using special tests.

Testing for epilepsy

If you are suspected of having epilepsy you may need tests or investigations. These will be used to:

1. Help decide whether or not you have epilepsy.
2. Help decide the kind of epilepsy, which is important in determining treatment.
3. Detect and diagnose a cause of the epilepsy.

EEG *investigations*

It is unusual for doctors to see someone having a seizure and equally unusual to be able to make an EEG recording during an attack, which is why a person's medical history and an eyewitness account always form the basis of a diagnosis. An EEG can be useful in adding more weight to a diagnosis of epilepsy and in classifying it. The EEG by itself is never enough to prove or disprove the diagnosis. Up to 10 per cent of people who have never had an epileptic fit have mildly abnormal electrical patterns and some people who have epilepsy have normal EEGs between their attacks. Still, since many people with epilepsy show abnormal EEG patterns between their attacks, this is a useful test.

An EEG is a very simple and painless procedure that should not cause you any stress or worry. We have seen that the brain

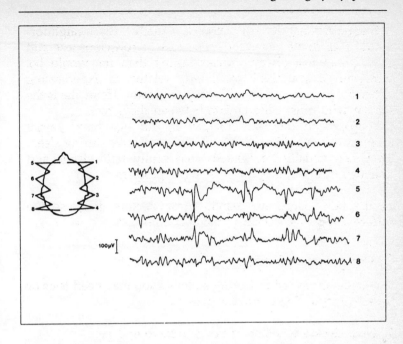

Typical spike discharges arising from the left side of the head. This person had a partial epilepsy.

works through networks of nerve cells that communicate with each other by electrical signals *(see page 6)*. The EEG detects and records this activity on paper or computer. It should not be confused with electroconvulsive therapy, when electricity is administered to the brain as a treatment for depression.

When you have an EEG, you will have approximately 20 metal tags lightly glued to your scalp. This allows up to 16 simultaneous recordings, or channels, from different parts of the brain. Sometimes the person's scalp is gently scratched beneath the tags to improve the recording. Because the electrical activity of the brain is difficult to detect and is easily obscured by any movement or muscle activity around the scalp, you will be asked to lie very still on a couch in a quiet environment. The recording takes about 20 to 30 minutes. At some point you might be asked to open and close your eyes, and to breathe deeply and regularly for a period of up to three

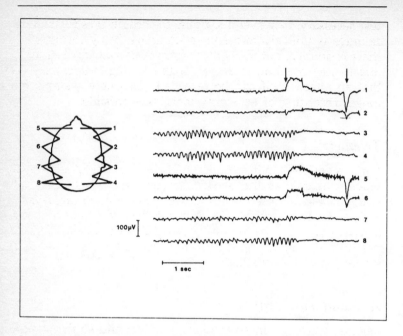

A normal eeg pattern. The regular activity in channels 3, 4, 7 and 8 is a normal alpha rhythm that occurs when someone lies still with closed eyes. The large waves marked by the arrows indicate eye movements, the first of which is associated with opening of the eyes, which abolishes the preceding alpha rhythm.

minutes. The technician might flash a strong light in your eyes. This is done to see if abnormal patterns are produced which would not otherwise be detected. If an abnormal pattern does develop, the technician will stop this part of the test to make sure that a seizure is not provoked. Sometimes EEGs are recorded during sleep, as particular kinds of epileptic abnormalities are more likely to occur then.

A normal EEG pattern is shown above. You can compare it with the abnormalities in the records from a person with a partial epilepsy *(see page 33)* and can compare both of them with abnormal records from people with generalized epilepsies *(see pages 24–25)*.

For most people with epilepsy, a standard EEG is the only

test necessary. However, recording the brainwaves for 20 to 30 minutes is unlikely to result in an attack being recorded. If there is doubt about the nature of someone's attacks and if the attacks are frequent, more prolonged testing is necessary so that an attack itself can be recorded. Two new systems for longer recording of EEGs now make this possible.

Telemetry

For this you remain in a room under constant observation by a video camera. At the same time an EEG is recorded on magnetic tape. These recordings can be continued for days at a time, so it is possible to compare the videotape of your activity with the pattern of EEG during an attack. This is particularly used to identify where seizures start in the brain if surgery is being considered.

Ambulatory monitoring

Telemetry is done in an artificial situation and so the results may still be ambiguous. A new system of ambulatory monitoring allows testing in more natural circumstances. It records 8–16 EEG channels on a portable tape recorder similar to a Walkman. After you have been into the recording unit to have the electrodes attached and the tape recorder turned on, you can leave the hospital and continue your normal routine. The tape can later be read with special equipment back at the hospital.

Imaging the brain

The last 20 years have seen enormous advances in the technologies that allow us to image the brain quite painlessly and without risk to people. Computerized tomography (CT) scanning and MR scanning are now readily available in most hospitals and every specialist centre. They now form an important part of the investigation of many people with epilepsy in order to detect damage and scarring, abnormalities of the development of the brain, abnormal blood vessels and, rarely, brain tumours, all of which may cause epilepsy.

CT scanning uses an X-ray beam to create images. You simply lie on a table and your head is placed in a specialized X-ray machine. The machine takes two-dimensional X-ray pictures of your head from a great many angles. The results are processed by a computer to produce an image of your brain, which shows considerable detail. CT scanning can show up a variety of cysts, scars and abnormal blood vessels in the brain, and can help identify the rare cases when people have some kind of tumour causing their epilepsy.

A new kind of scanning that has become very important for people with epilepsy is magnetic resonance imaging (MRI). This is a revolutionary new technique in which a person lies with his or her head within a large, very powerful circular magnet. Images are produced by changes in the magnetic field which are analysed by a computer used to construct images of the brain. No X-rays are involved in this technique and it produces very high quality pictures.

This form of scanning is now available for people with epilepsy attending specialist neurology and epilepsy centres. It shows up minor scarring, developmental abnormalities and some forms of tumours much better than does CT scanning. It is essential for anyone considering surgical treatment.

Blood tests are less helpful. They can be used to detect low blood sugar, low blood calcium, and evidence of infection and kidney or liver failure, but they are not necessary for most people. Anyone whose epilepsy is caused by one of these problems will probably have many complaints other than just seizures and so will have to have a series of thorough tests.

Is retesting ever necessary?

Once initial tests have been completed, it is not often necessary to have repeat tests. Occasionally further EEGs are helpful, if:

- treatment is not being as effective as expected
- new symptoms develop
- stopping drug treatment is being considered

In the next chapter we describe the different types of

treatment available and which you are most likely to be given according to the sort of seizures you have. We also talk about the chances of doing without drugs after a period of treatment – when and for whom this is possible.

Section II

Living with Epilepsy

5

A personal view
by Sue Usiskin

The Beginning

At 15 the school art studio was the place I most loved to be. In retrospect, it seems strange that my epilepsy started there. As I sat at my easel, absorbed by my painting, my eyes suddenly locked. This odd sensation intensified and my head began to jerk of its own accord. I heard my paintbrush land on the boarded floor. I tried to call out but could not make any sound. I fell backwards off my chair. There was a loud crash, then blackness and silence.

We lived about 30 minutes from the school by car, so I was puzzled to see my parents leaning over me as I opened my eyes. My head throbbed and there were cuts on the backs of my hands. The studio was very quiet.

'Well, I'll be going now,' said an unfamiliar voice.

I turned my face in its direction to find the school doctor closing her bag. By her side stood the headmistress with a look of concern on her face. I was surprised to see her in the art studio; it was not a place she usually visited! My parents took me home to bed where our family doctor came to see me. He checked my reflexes and my balance and we talked about what had happened to me. He suggested that I should see a specialist and an appointment was made for the following week. We were ushered into the waiting room. I flicked through the pile of magazines with clammy, nervous hands. The silence was punctuated only by the ticking of the wall clock.

'The doctor will see you now,' said a voice from the corridor.

We rose from our chairs and entered the consulting room.

The doctor rose, extending his hand to my parents. After the introductions, we sat down and he took notes on my general health and asked questions about my family history. He was fairly certain that what I had experienced in the art studio the previous week was an epileptic seizure, or fit. I would have to undergo a few tests at the hospital, after which he would see us again. He said that the treatment for my condition was 'not to have it', which puzzled me.

He explained that he felt that I had had an epileptic seizure and would need an EEG before this could be confirmed. Once the diagnosis was known it would be possible to control the seizures with medication which he would prescribe.

'What is an EEG? I don't think I know.'

'It's short for electroencephalogram, which means a tracing of the impulses given out by the brain. Certain patterns tell us if there are problems and which areas of the brain they come from. Just stand up for me, will you?' he asked. 'Now, I want you to follow my finger with your left eye, keeping the other eye covered. Good. Now the other side.'

He continued his instructions and after about five minutes he told me to sit down again. Returning to his desk, he made a number of notes while I shifted in my chair in nervous anticipation.

The tests would be done on Friday morning and the results available the following week. He would also be writing to our GP and the school and would like to see us again in a week's time.

A few days later I went to have the eeg and a technician attached a number of electrodes to my scalp with long wires. I must have looked rather like an astronaut! The whole process was entirely painless and quickly over. When we returned to see the doctor the following week he told my parents that he had seen the EEG results and felt it would be a good idea to begin my treatment immediately. He explained that it would take time for me to adjust to the anti-epileptic drugs. In the event of any difficulty, I was to contact him.

Adjustments and side-effects

It was, in fact, nine months before I had another seizure. I remember very little about this period of my life, mainly because the anti-epileptic regime that he prescribed made me feel vague and sleepy much of the time. The second seizure also happened at school. After I had recovered sufficiently to be moved down to the sick room, I was lying wondering how often this was going to happen when I heard the familiar voice of my class teacher.

'I thought we had finished with all this,' she said.

I was to learn that there are apparently no limits to what people will say if they are ignorant about epilepsy.

Once again my parents were asked to come and collect me. I slept most of that day, waking only in order to take my anti-epileptic medication. I contacted my specialist who suggested a slight increase in my medication and the addition of another drug to give better control of my seizures.

I began to feel increasingly drowsy with the additions to my medication. No amount of sleep made any difference. I expressed my concern but was told that I should continue the medication and my body would adjust in time. It didn't. I found myself living in the twilight world of sedation and I still had seizures from time to time. I have very little idea of how different my life would have been at that time had there been available the plasma level tests that today so efficiently measure the concentrations of medication in the blood. Since the advent of these tests, I have never again had to endure the misery of drug intoxication.

Up to that time I had had a great many friends, both at school and socially, but now I became increasingly selective about the company I kept. My father saw it as a way of protecting myself – by getting out of social relationships first, I was sparing myself the pain of rejection by others should they find it difficult to cope with my unpredictable condition. My first major seizure in public consolidated my fears of rejection.

One evening I was waiting for a bus with my friends when I had a seizure. Afterwards I thought that being seen with me when I was having a seizure might be a problem for them, as they might feel that it somehow reflected on them. Mid adolescence is a time of acute self-consciousness and so the prospect of being seen with someone who suddenly collapses on the ground in a noisy, jerking heap was one pressure they could do without. Thus my social relationships became fewer and the consequent isolation aroused within me a sense of being different.

Until then, the relationship between my parents and siblings was good, however the onset of my epilepsy and need for extra support were unsettling for the rest of the family, who began to compete for attention in various ways. Just as my parents had been called to school in connection with my health, they were now being called to discuss emotional problems with my two sisters' teachers. They did not realize there was any connection between my own needs and those of my sisters and brother.

My parents coped admirably with all the adjustments that these initial few years brought. They never tried to limit my activities because of what people might think if I had a fit, which would have been all too easy to do and would, I am sure, have saved them many anxious moments. I was fortunate that they were not overprotective and I was not made to feel delicate or incapable. On the contrary, they realized that I needed to do more than accept my epilepsy if I was to develop into an integrated member of society. I was encouraged to make an extra effort to overcome my difficulties and not to allow them to become an excuse for doing less. In any long-term condition, it is vital to develop a positive attitude. If this is not fostered from the start, it becomes increasingly difficult to develop later. It is most important to have a coping strategy to be able to share with others, so they can take their cue from you. This is not always easy to achieve, but improves with experience.

My school work began to suffer. The medication had severely reduced my ability to concentrate and I took a very long time to complete my homework every night. I would sit at my desk for hours, struggling to apply myself and finishing only a modest amount. Sometimes the effect was such that I would stare out of the bedroom window in a daze, stirring only at the sound of my mother's voice calling me to come down for supper. Despite these difficulties I managed to obtain seven GCSE passes with reasonable grades. I did well in art, which had always been my best subject and the one I wished to pursue.

College days

My mother was a sculptor specializing in the human form. With this background it seemed natural that I should now apply to art college. I was delighted to hear that I had been accepted. My boyfriend was studying at the same art college and we both belonged to an amateur drama group in our spare time. I had heard that in some cases spotlights act as a trigger in epilepsy and I think it was then that I had to make my first conscious decision about how my condition should affect my life in general. I used practical danger as my yardstick. If an activity put me in real physical danger, I would not risk it. For example, I loved riding horses, but I thought the chance of having an epileptic attack while doing so was not worth the risk. However, I did not believe that spotlights constituted a comparable danger so did not avoid activities such as the drama group.

The last 18 months had been important to me socially. I had begun to evaluate my health and realized that generally I remained quite healthy. This was a boost to my hitherto sagging self-confidence. It is true that 'nothing succeeds like success' and although I was still having seizures, I was beginning to live with my epilepsy. I had been happy to discover that my condition did not appear to discourage boyfriends, as I had feared; on the contrary, they were satisfied with a simple explanation and some practical tips. Maybe they felt protective towards me. All I knew was they did not seem overtly concerned by my revelation. My parents were obviously delighted by my refound gregarious personality and suggested that I give a party for my friends. I had been to many parties over the past months and this would be an opportunity to return some of the invitations. I was grateful for their suggestion and enjoyed the occasion with real enthusiasm.

While I was at college I became aware for the first time of just how other people saw epilepsy, when I was called upon to help when a fellow student had a seizure in the college canteen one afternoon. As I looked down at her rigidly convulsing body, which was emitting strange grunting sounds, I could understand why it could be frightening. I had never realized how undignified a seizure could be and I found it hard to identify with what I witnessed. I was sure it was this, combined with epilepsy's unpredictable nature, that other people found difficult to cope with. A seizure may happen at any time, anywhere, which gives it a high nuisance value for you as well as for the onlooker. Never knowing when your next seizure will strike makes it very difficult to plan ahead, but no matter how hard you try to live from day to day, a certain amount of planning is necessary and desirable. If you do have to drop out of something, you have to accept the fact and try to replan the activity for another time. It is highly unlikely that you will have to cancel the same thing twice.

Living on my own

I enjoyed my years at art college very much indeed. After one year on the foundation course, I applied to a degree course at another college. To my delight, I was accepted and began to plan for the changes. It was to be the first of many changes in my life. I had been thinking about moving out of my family home, as I needed to be able to work uninterrupted and without disturbing anyone else. The only time I found I could do this was quite late in the evening when no one else was about. I would still be working in the small hours of the morning, completely absorbed by whatever I was doing. My bedroom was very small and I needed more space to spread out while working on a variety of design projects. I began to look for a place that would provide me with the extra space and my first opportunity to live on my own.

Eventually I found what I was looking for. With the help and encouragement of my parents, despite any reservations that they must have had, I moved into a small terraced cottage. It seemed to be ideal, providing a room where I could work downstairs and a bed-sitting room upstairs. My parents agreed to the proposed move and helped me to organize it. The encouragement they gave me at this time was remarkable considering how concerned they must have been about my living alone. However they felt, they supported my move with enthusiasm. I was extremely lucky. Their positive attitude enabled me to function at 19 as an independent young adult, with sufficient confidence not to hide behind my health problem. I did not fully appreciate just how important this was until I met one of my neighbours.

One day while searching for my keys, I was greeted by a new neighbour who was quite out of breath. She introduced herself, saying that she lived on my right with her husband and two daughters, then asked me to excuse her, as her elder daughter was at home not feeling well. Next time we met I asked how her daughter was feeling and learned why she was not at work once more. 'She's had one of her turns again,' explained her mother. 'It's such a shame, she's had rather a lot lately.'

It soon became clear to me that the girl had epilepsy. Her mother was embarrassed about it, so she referred to it as 'turns', a euphemism I have often heard. Many people find they cannot get the word 'epilepsy' past their lips. Although we have come a long way since the time when 'epileptics' were thought to be possessed by the devil and burned at the stake as witches, prejudice lingers on. The idea that epilepsy is a form of insanity still exists and many people are very guarded about the condition, which is understandable.

Eventually, I met my neighbour's daughter. She was extremely shy and withdrawn. It was clear that she had a profound sense of being different, but it was quite different from mine – there emanated from her an air of shame. As I got to know the family better I saw that there was a definite link between her parents' inability to accept her condition and the way she coped with it. Their overprotection meant that she had missed the opportunity to develop a positive attitude to her life and to emerge as a confident adult.

The years I spent at college while living on my own were very happy ones. I always felt content at home. I was often asked if I missed company and I would reply that as I worked with other people all day, I rather enjoyed being alone at night. I saw my friends and family when I wanted to and it seemed a perfect arrangement. I worked hard, but was still having problems with the side-effects of my anti-epileptic drugs, which were affecting my concentration. There were times when I felt thoroughly depressed, for although I was grateful for the measure of control over my seizures that the drugs afforded, it seemed to me a high price to pay in terms of dulled energy. My specialist did not appear to be concerned about this and even suggested I take a mild tranquillizer in addition to my other drugs to stop me worrying about the side-effects! He assured me that this other drug he was prescribing also had anti-epileptic properties and therefore might give a better degree of control over my seizures. I felt cornered. My instincts told me that the present 'cocktail' was sufficient, not to say excessive, but it had never given me the complete control I had hoped for. After much deliberation I agreed to try, but only because at the time I felt I was in no position to refuse. I wanted to be able to control my epilepsy.

During my last year at college I began to see a lot more of my boyfriend Andrew. I had completed a collection of designs that I hoped to market and he encouraged me to start work as a freelance fashion designer. My plan was eventually to set up a small fashion accessory business that I could run from home. It seemed to be a practical way of coping with my unpredictable health problem, as it meant I did not have to travel. I had been put off using the underground when one day I felt a seizure start whilst going down a steep, crowded escalator at an underground station. It was the rush hour and I was packed in the crowd like the proverbial sardine in a tin. I found myself unable to move, locked firmly between the people standing in front of and behind me. In this way I was prevented from falling down the length of the escalator. I had always hated crowds, but I realized then that they had their uses after all! Thereafter I reduced travelling to an absolute minimum. Escalators, along with riding and climbing, were 'not worth the risk'.

Marriage, pregnancy and medication

Whenever my epilepsy gave particular cause for concern I would tell my specialist, whose response would be to increase my medication, sometimes prescribing additional drugs without monitoring their effect. It is no surprise that this way of dealing with my epilepsy proved to be disastrous. My health suffered and it was not long before my condition had deteriorated markedly and I began to feel vacant and lethargic. Although it was difficult for me, I someone managed to continue to run my small business from home, encouraged by Andrew.

He had established a design business of his own, which he operated from a studio about two miles away. My family were very fond of him and delighted when they heard that we wanted to get married the following year.

We both wanted to have children and thought it would be a good idea to talk to my doctor about the hereditary aspects of epilepsy. He said I had a 10 per cent chance of passing it on to our children. Andrew and I took the view that such a relatively small chance was worth taking. In any case, I continued to live with my epilepsy and saw no reason why, should the need arise, we could not help a child to do the same.

When I became pregnant, Andrew suggested that it would be best for me to attend the obstetric clinic at the same hospital where I was seen for my epilepsy as I was very worried about the effect of my frequent attacks on our unborn child. I was never warned of the effects my drugs could have on the baby. Happily, apart from being a month premature, our son, Oliver, was unaffected.

My seizures were very frequent at that time and I depended on Andrew for practical help when the baby arrived. He encouraged me to seek a second opinion. Looking back, I realize that if it had not been for his support, I might still be taking excessive doses of anti-epileptic drugs, unaware of any alternative.

The first thing my new specialist discovered was that I was grossly intoxicated by the anti-epileptic medication I had been given over the years in ever-increasing amounts. In his opinion I was having more seizures because I was so run down by the treatment I had been receiving. Gradually this was simplified and reduced. I began to feel alive again and my condition improved from having up to three seizures a day to about three a month.

Now I was able to look after Oliver. I was extremely disappointed that I could not breast feed him. I was told that the drugs I was taking would have affected my milk. They are not given nowadays. Andrew shared the bottle feeds with me, which meant that I got sufficient sleep. My approach was always practical. I never bathed Oliver when I was alone with him. This safety precaution was one that I applied to myself as well, in case of an attack, and adhere to still. I also doubled up on changing equipment to avoid having to carry the baby repeatedly up and down the stairs, and I changed him while he lay on a mat on the floor rather than on a bed from which he might fall if I had an attack. Apart from these precautions, I set about caring for Oliver in just the same way as any other young mother.

We also took safety measures in the kitchen to minimize any risks. Though to date I have not had an accident while cooking, I always use casserole-style saucepans, without long handles, because if I were to have an attack near the cooker I would be less likely to knock them over. Similarly, I have never used an eye-level grill, as during an attack it would be easy to pull the grill pan out too far and spill its contents over myself and others. My personal rule is never to cook on gas because of all the dangers that naked flames could bring.

I was delighted with the reduction in my seizures. The connection between the level of my medication and my condition was undeniable. The new specialist explained to us that it is possible to poison a person by exceeding a correct level of drugs in his or her blood. Toxins accumulate in this way and lead to other problems, such as the ones I had experienced. I was very grateful for his help.

It was not long before Oliver could pull himself up in his cot and our thoughts turned to finding accommodation that was slightly larger. Andrew could run his business from anywhere, providing he had a telephone, a desk and a drawing board, and he thought it would be a good idea if he were on hand in case I needed him. We eventually found a home with the space we needed. It was a great source of strength for me to know that Andrew was near and there were many times when his help was really useful.

Helping the children to cope

As soon as Oliver was mobile we realized that he would need help to cope with my epilepsy. We found the best way was to give him a small task to perform while I was having a seizure.

His contribution was to get a cloth to place under my face to absorb any saliva produced and at the same time prevent me from grazing myself as I lay there. In a very short time he was able to 'help Mummy' whenever the need arose. However, it was not so simple when we were out.

It seemed that however well Oliver was able to cope at home, as soon as we were out the odds were stacked against us. Most people are quite ignorant about epilepsy and so the reaction to a fit is often unhelpful to say the least. When Oliver was about two years old, I had a seizure in a taxi. The driver took one look and yelled, 'Get out of my cab! Go on, get out. I'm not having any drunks in my cab.'

It was raining hard, but he opened the door and dragged me out, leaving me to have the fit in the wet street accompanied by a sobbing toddler. This kind of incident was bound to leave its mark on Oliver, however well adjusted he seemed in other circumstances. We persevered, hoping that by giving him a framework within which to cope he would eventually grow in confidence.

During my first pregnancy I had still been taking large debilitating doses of various anti-epileptic drugs, so it was a relief when I became pregnant again to find that I suffered infinitely fewer seizures than before. None the less, the birth of our daughter marked the beginning of an intensely traumatic few years for both of us.

Anna was born with a congenital heart defect. When it was diagnosed, no indication could be given about her future and as she looked terribly ill at this stage we were very anxious. I am sure that in addition to a mother's instinct to do everything to help her child I was able to bring another dimension to her life. I knew from my own experience how crucial the attitude of the parents can be in building up sufficient confidence in a child to make life as normal as possible and prevent him or her feeling isolated and inadequate. Andrew was marvellously supportive and his strength and positive attitude were key elements in Anna's progress. To the surprise and delight of the doctors, Anna had recovered considerably by the time she was three.

When they were small, Oliver and Anna played games together like many young children. A favourite for them both was mummies and daddies. Anna was directed in her role as Mummy by her brother. Oliver's list of instructions was a source of great amusement to us. He would say, 'Anna, you're going shopping.'

Anna obligingly responded by carrying a shopping bag across the room.

'Now you go to buy some bread.'

Anna mimed buying bread and putting her purchase in the bag.

'Now you have a seizure!'

At this command Anna's shopping expedition would stop. She dropped to the floor and proceeded to imitate my convulsions. There was a lot of shaking and groaning, accompanied by ample spitting. After this she would lie still until Oliver told her to get up and continue her shopping. They continued to play together in this way for many years and I am convinced that it helped them come to terms with my condition, which could otherwise have had a very inhibiting effect on them both.

When I think of some of the distressing situations we have lived through as a direct result of my epilepsy, I cannot help feeling amazed at my family's resilience. One afternoon when Anna was about three years old, we were walking down the busy high street to meet Oliver from school when I began to have a seizure. In the confusion that must have followed poor Anna was left stranded in the street watching me being whisked away by an ambulance that had been sent for by a well-meaning passer-by. No one had noticed her in the crowd and she tearfully made her way to Oliver's school, knowing that there would be nobody to meet him. Fortunately, when she arrived someone took care of her, but this kind of experience had an unsettling effect on us all. Afterwards, she woke up twice nightly for six months just to make sure I was still there.

Out in public

I make a point of telling people I come into regular contact with about my epilepsy. I feel more at ease with people who know what to expect and they are grateful for the opportunity to ask me how best to help. Many people do not realize, for example, that it takes quite a while until I am able to speak again after an attack. If we have discussed this point beforehand, they will be prepared for it. However, attacks do occur in public when there is no familiar face to put me at my ease and this can present problems.

I sometimes get a warning that an attack is imminent and then I try to get to a safe place at once. The first sign of a seizure in my case is that my eyes fix on something. I know that from the moment this happens I have just a few seconds until the attack is in full force. The next stage of the warning is a jerking of my eyes to one side, closely followed by my head and neck. I have trained myself to use this short time to get down flat in the least cluttered space – away from walls, furniture and sharp objects – in order to avoid injury.

On one occasion, I was passing a large post office when I felt unwell. I went inside and made my way past the long queue to where the staff were. I tried to attract their attention by tapping on the glass door marked Staff Only. I was feeling increasingly unwell when a young man came towards me from behind the counter.

'Can't you read?' he demanded curtly. 'Staff Only!'

'Yes,' I said weakly, 'but I have epilepsy and I feel unwell.' I got out my official epilepsy card, which I carry with me at all times, to show him. 'I just want to sit down quietly . . .' I began to explain.

'Then why don't you go back out on the street where you belong?' came the retort. With that he simply turned on his heel and walked away.

This kind of response is, of course, a result of ignorance and the fear that accompanies it. Fortunately, I have also encountered people who are kind and helpful.

One fine spring day I was walking towards our local shops when I felt the first signs of an attack. There was no one in sight as I lay down on the pavement, trying to cradle my head in my arms. I heard a vehicle braking sharply near by, followed by quick footsteps. The attack gained momentum and as it did I became aware of someone kneeling over me.

'It's okay, love,' he said. 'I'll wait with you.'

Some time elapsed and as the seizure neared its final phase, the young man assured me that I was all right and must not worry. I lay in a daze on the pavement until he suggested that I might be more comfortable if I sat in his van for a while. I looked around for my handbag, still feeling dazed as he helped me to my feet. It certainly was more comfortable sitting in the van. The young man now assured me that he was not in a hurry and would wait with me until I felt well enough to go home. He seemed genuinely concerned for my welfare and his kind, gentle manner put me at my ease.

When I felt a little better, he offered to drive me home, I am not in the habit of accepting lifts from strangers, but this young man's caring manner filled me with confidence. He drove the half mile to my home and helped me down from his van.

'Hope you feel better soon,' he called as he turned to go.

On various other occasions I have derived quite a bit of amusement from the things people say while I'm having an attack. Unless I lose consciousness, I can hear what is going on around me. I realize that to many people the fact that the children are so calm and practical while their mother is out of control is in itself difficult to grasp. For Oliver and Anna the most pressing task is to try to persuade them that it is not the first time I have had a seizure, that I will recover and that there is no need to send for an ambulance. Quite how loath people are to believe what a child says in this sort of situation is clearly demonstrated by the following story.

I was in the local butcher's shop when I had a seizure. Oliver was kneeling down in the sawdust trying to look after me when I heard a customer say, 'Does mother often do this?'

When his reply was affirmative she became quite indignant. 'Really? Are you sure?' as if he were trying to lead her on! To this woman it was utterly unbelievable – not only was I shaking, groaning and foaming on the floor but, according to my son, I did it often.

There have been times when I feel that my condition has imposed a considerable burden on my children. It is easy to attribute more or less all the emotional difficulties that my growing children experience to my health. One has to be aware of certain things that can be linked firmly to living with epilepsy. Both Oliver and Anna have gone through periods when they have repeatedly asked me how I am. It is not surprising, as they know only too well the risky nature of my life. It would be surprising if they showed no concern and the fact that they do not make a secret of it can only be good.

One day I was walking to the shops on a particularly wet and wintry afternoon when I felt the first signs of a seizure. I leaned heavily against the glass of the nearest shop, a building society. Beckoning for help, I crumpled slowly to the floor as I entered. I felt very conspicuous as, apart from myself, the shop was empty. The staff stayed exactly where they were behind the counter.

As the seizure ended, I wondered how I might get one of the staff to call Andrew, who had moved to a local office since both children were now at school. I fumbled in my bag and managed to retrieve my card with his number on it. When Andrew arrived, the staff, still behind the counter, explained that they thought I was the 'front', the diversion, for a robbery and had they come to my aid an accomplice would have got behind the counter. I sat on the floor in complete disbelief. Andrew explained that my condition was quite genuine. The manager told us that he couldn't take any risks and he seemed adamant about it.

I always try, whenever possible, to overcome the ignorance with education. The following day I put a leaflet about first aid for seizures through their letter flap in the hope that their response might, in future, be different.

At times it is easy to lose faith in human nature and it is encouraging to recall this incident, which took place in a Marks & Spencer store. As I was wheeling a trolley through the food department I began to feel unwell. I approached a member of staff and said, 'I have epilepsy and I do not feel well.'

'Don't you worry, love. I'll help you,' he assured me. As he spoke he gently helped me down to the floor.

When the attack had ended, the staff helped me into a wheelchair and I was taken to their recovery room, where I could lie down in peace. As soon as I was ready, they helped me down to the street.

I wrote to Marks & Spencer describing the way their staff

had coped. If more companies could learn from their excellent example, then people with epilepsy would have a far easier time.

Unfortunately, some people have a mistaken idea of what to do and on one occasion I had a seizure when I heard someone say, 'You have to pull out her tongue and hang on to it while you slap her around the face.'

I was horrified and tried to prevent this imminent assault. As my assailant leaned over me, I summoned up all my strength and kicked her. At the same time I made as much noise as possible in the hope that she would take the hint. She did. The experience probably confirmed all her worst fears about people with epilepsy, but I had to defend myself.

Injury

One of the worst aspects of living with epilepsy is that you injure yourself quite often. This is most likely to happen in the street, a singularly unsympathetic place for a seizure. Usually the damage is quite minor. The bruises and grazes look a lot worse than they really are, but it is still depressing to have a visible reminder of an unpleasant event. Every year, thousands of accidents occur at home and good safety precautions are important if your epilepsy is not well controlled by medication. A full description of the precautions you can take is given on page 98.

Prejudice and Education

Many people with epilepsy complain of prejudice and certainly living with epilepsy is not made any easier as a result. I always ask myself how much I really knew about the condition before I was diagnosed myself and whether I may have held some of the strange views about epilepsy that are born of ignorance before I knew any different.

Someone once said that I must be grateful to Andrew for marrying me as he did not think many people would want to marry someone with epilepsy. I explained that we led a normal life – punctuated by seizures – and saw no reason to be grateful in the sense that he implied.

The answer to prejudice is education. Young people need to grow up better informed of health matters and a compulsory course of first aid together with a broad education would be an advantage. Videotapes and slides could be used, and could form the basis for discussions. This would go a long way towards removing ignorance and fear, and so promote greater understanding and tolerance. My involvement with health education and epilepsy has been a priority and remains so.

Living with epilepsy helps keep things in proportion. While it is often a source of stress, it can be a means of uniting and strengthening family relationships. It can help one keep a balanced perspective on life and not take things for granted. In a school essay titled 'Relatives and how to cope with them', Oliver wrote:

My Mum has a thing called epilepsy, in other words epileptic fits. Every month or so she has them. It is hard to see your own mother lying on the ground shaking and foaming at the mouth but I have found that, hard as it is, just think how lucky you are it is not you. I know I have lots of things to worry about but I have learnt how to cope with them, so I'm not that unlucky.

When I read this, I was encouraged to find that Oliver was able to see things in such a mature way at his young age.

Today, much can be done to help people with epilepsy. About 75 per cent will eventually achieve complete control on their medication, while 25 per cent may have to live with active seizures. The latter group in particular may encounter some problems adapting to the condition which may not be dealt with in a hospital clinic. A doctor may not realize that an anxious patient may be unable to absorb much information. Repeated interviews are often necessary to deal with such issues as fear, anger, denial and confusion. Continuity of care is important in establishing good communication and a feeling of trust.

People often have misconceptions about their epilepsy which they find difficult to introduce into a conversation with their doctor or counsellor. These include the association of epilepsy with mental disorders, presumed inheritance and the effect of seizures. It is important to discuss these aspects openly so that patients do not add to the burden of their condition. An experienced counsellor, familiar with the difficulties people with epilepsy may suffer with their careers, social lives, family relationships and self-esteem, can have much to offer. He or she can address problems, give accurate information and support. The use of coping strategies to help build confidence and a positive attitude will help lower anxiety and improve quality of life. Epilepsy is more than a medical diagnosis and may influence many aspects of life. Concern may increase at particular times, such as starting school or work, living on your own or becoming a parent, and it is not uncommon to experience a wide range of emotions. It is helpful to talk over your feelings and begin to look objectively at your situation. The diagnosis of epilepsy may have a direct impact on you and those around you are also affected and may react in different ways. It is important to talk about your feelings and not hide them.

Living with epilepsy is often trying. Your attitude is important and can influence how you feel about yourself and how others see you. Try to concentrate on the things that you can do rather than those you can't. We hope that this book will help you explore what you can do to manage your epilepsy by playing an active rather than a passive role.

6

Epilepsy: from babyhood to old age

Having epilepsy is going to affect your everyday life but it should not make an as enormous a difference as you may at first think. Some commonsense precautions may be needed, but there is no need to deprive yourself unnecessarily of doing things. Obviously, everyone who has epilepsy is different and what may be risky for one person may be perfectly acceptable for another. In this chapter we give advice that we hope will be useful in helping you adapt to a lifestyle that is best for you as an individual. As a starting-point, the table below lists guidelines that apply to everyone.

Having epilepsy has different implications depending on the type of epilepsy you have (*see pages 24–40*) and the age when the condition first appeared. In this chapter we discuss the worries many people have about how their epilepsy may affect them at different stages in their lives, both emotionally and physically.

Practical Guidelines for Living with Epilepsy

Do

- Ask for information and advice about your epilepsy and its treatment.

- Make the most of your talents.

- Consider carefully the risks to yourself and other people of undertaking specific activities. If in doubt, ask advice, but try to err on the side of living a full and active life.

- Take your medication regularly and as directed.

- Avoid specific circumstances that might make your fits more likely.

- Try to talk to people about your epilepsy and correct their misconceptions.

- Consider joining one of the epilepsy associations. They might be able to offer you help and you might be able to help others.

- Consider helping with research into epilepsy either by taking part in clinical trials or by helping to raise money.

Don't

- Remain in ignorance.

- Use epilepsy as an excuse for not realizing your potential.

- Miss doses or take extra doses when you 'don't feel well'.

- Drink heavily or have too many late nights in a row.

- Keep teachers or employers in ignorance of your epilepsy.

Family life

Naturally everyone in the family is going to be affected by one of you having epilepsy.

Children

Bear in mind the advice throughout this book, that you should lead as normal a life as possible, and this means that the person with epilepsy should not expect special treatment and overprotection from relatives. Children with epilepsy should be treated in the same way as any brother or sister. Their independence should be encouraged as far as is reasonable and they must follow the usual rules, particularly if there are other children in the family. Make as few allowances for epilepsy as possible and don't allow it to be used as a means of manipulation – that will only cause greater long-term tensions within the family and problems of getting along with others for the person concerned.

Babies and young children

Having a baby diagnosed as having epilepsy will be upsetting for both parents. What you should never do is feel guilty about the condition having developed. No one is responsible for his or her genetic make-up. Brain damage caused at birth can be blamed on any number of reasons. It is futile and damaging for the whole family to spend time agonizing over these issues. The best thing for you and your baby is to establish as soon as you can a smooth-running routine following your doctor's instructions on giving medication, and coping with fits and minimum upset and fuss.

How much protection should you give?
We believe you should avoid restraint as much as possible. For a toddler or older child having sudden and unpredictable fits which result in falls, a head protector may be necessary. These are lightweight and designed to be as uncumbersome as possible.

Obviously there is a need for more supervision than with most children, and as your child grows and begins walking you will have to stop anything too dangerous such as climbing. Nevertheless, you must let your child explore his or her environment as much as possible as this is so important in learning and development.

Can you anticipate a seizure?
This is difficult unless there are certain triggers that have been identified, or your baby has febrile seizures *(see page 36)*. Then you can avoid a fever by keeping the baby's temperature down with tepid sponging.

When do you explain the condition?

To your child
As soon as you think your child can begin to understand. This is best not only because adjustment is easier if knowledge comes as naturally as possible, but also because your child

will need to understand why regular medicine is necessary. Children should be encouraged to take their own medicine – under sensible supervision.

To friends and relatives
Again, as soon as possible. This is particularly important for anyone who will be taking responsibility for your child at any time.

Schooling

At one time all children with epilepsy were considered seriously disabled and were educated in special schools. Now it is recognized that only a small number of children need to go to special schools, either because their seizures are so difficult to control or because they also suffer from other physical disabilities, or learning or behavioural problems. (The names and addresses of schools with specific facilities for children with epilepsy are listed on page 139.)

If it has been decided that your child can continue to attend an ordinary school, your first priority must be to tell the teachers about the epilepsy. You must be completely frank in discussing the condition with the teachers – they are no more likely to be well informed about epilepsy than anyone else who has no previous experience of it. All the teachers in the school must be aware that your child has epilepsy. They need to know what might happen during a fit and what action to take *(see page 22)*.

If a seizure does happen at school, once the fit itself has subsided the teacher in charge should take your child to a quiet area to allow peaceful recovery. It is hardly ever necessary to send a child with epilepsy home. The school staff should be told about the medicine the doctor has prescribed and whether they need to supervise a midday dose. If possible, of course, your child should take medication at home in the morning before going to school and in the evening after returning home. This is possible for almost all anti-epileptic drugs and is much better than taking tablets into school.

You must emphasize that the school should avoid identifying your child as being different from the other children. He or she must obey the school rules just the same as the rest of the children and should take part in the fullest range of activities possible. Most children can take part in physical education, including sports and swimming, as long as the teacher in charge can provide enough supervision to cover any eventualities such as a possible fit. Your doctor will advise you about how much your child can and should do. It may be wise for children with epilepsy not to participate in climbing activities.

Ultimately, the care of your child and the activities undertaken during school hours will be the responsibility of the school staff. You, the parents, should be in regular contact so that you can discuss with the teachers any problems resulting from your child's epilepsy. Whenever any of you is uncertain as to the correct course of action, you must seek advice from the doctor supervising your child. Schooling should be an enjoyable experience and one that will develop your child's talents to the full.

Adolescence

Adolescence is usually the time when people develop their independence and start to take responsibility for their own life. It is a time when relationships with people outside the family become more important. Having epilepsy can make these always difficult processes even more difficult and everyone in the family needs to appreciate this.

Will you have changing patterns of attacks?
Seizures may change during adolescence. Petit mal seizures tend to become less frequent and children who have had these sometimes start to experience tonic-clonic seizures. Children with brain damage and symptomatic generalized epilepsy may start to have more classical complex partial seizures during the teenage years (*see page 47*). Other influences that could bring on more attacks are the classic triggers: too little sleep and too much alcohol!

If you have just been diagnosed and are coping with the physical and emotional tensions everyone experiences in adolescence, having epilepsy may seem an impossible burden.

You may be tempted to rebel against your condition and ignore medication and visits to your doctor. You won't be in a mood to welcome good advice. Nevertheless, this is not a time to withdraw into your shell. It will be much easier to live with your epilepsy if you can talk about it openly:

● Do find a doctor you feel you can communicate with.
● Do tell your friends about your condition and how to help you during a seizure.
● Don't restrict your life. Follow your favourite pursuits – within reason. You will find there are surprisingly few that you can't enjoy.

Going to college

A lot of people with epilepsy go on to higher education. If you have won a place at a college or university you will need to make a few special preparations.

Tell the college medical officer and your own tutor that you have epilepsy.

If possible, arrange to live in a hall of residence, at least for the first part of your course. This means you won't have to bother with cooking and domestic chores while you become used to the new lifestyle. You will also have plenty of contact with other students and know there are always people to help during a seizure.

All examiners, internal and external, should be informed that you have epilepsy. They may need to make allowances for this when marking your papers, should a fit have occurred during an examination.

Does too much studying bring on a seizure?
I don't believe this ever happens. But you must avoid falling into the trap of studying late at night. Lack of sleep certainly brings on seizures.

Personal and sexual relationships

Some people with epilepsy do experience difficulty in getting along with schoolmates, friends and workmates – but so do many people who do not have epilepsy. The question that always arises is: whom should you tell that you have epilepsy? Often people are secretive about their epilepsy because they feel that it will alter people's attitudes towards them. Unfortunately, this can happen, but secrecy almost certainly perpetuates the myths and misunderstandings that surround epilepsy, so that in the long term it is the wrong choice. The more people who realize that one of their friends, their teacher, a workmate, has epilepsy and is still a very able and active member of society, the less prejudice there is likely to be about it.

The ultimate test of anyone's success in forming personal relationships is likely to be marriage and family life. People with epilepsy can marry and bring up children with the same hope of success as anyone else. But the potential worries about contraception, pregnancy and inheritance are among the most frequent we hear about at our clinics.

Contraception

The oral contraceptive pill is still the most convenient and effective method of contraception for women with epilepsy. If you are used to taking medication, you are unlikely to forget the pill, and its success rate as a contraceptive is still high. However, certain anti-epileptic drugs – phenytoin, carbamazepine and phenobarbitone – affect the body's metabolism. This means that the active substances in the pill, the oestrogen hormones, are made inactive more quickly and efficiently than they would be otherwise. Very rarely this can result in unwanted pregnancies.

Most standard pills contain very low levels of oestrogen. If you experience bleeding between periods, which is a clear indication that not enough oestrogen is being taken into the body, you will need to take pills with a higher levels of oestrogen to maintain the right level for effective contraception. Discuss this with your doctor or family planning clinic, who can make sure that you are taking the right strength of pill. Higher strength pills do not carry any additional risks for women with epilepsy. There is no evidence that taking the pill makes seizures better or worse.

There is increasing resistance to the pill because of possible, very small, increases in the risks of heart disease or cancer. If you feel unhappy about taking the pill, you can use one of the other means of contraception that are satisfactory for people with epilepsy. Your doctor or family planning clinic can advise you on what is best for you as an individual.

Pregnancy

What is the risk of having a child with epilepsy?
Overall, two to three people in every 100 will have epilepsy during their lives. If a parent has epilepsy the risks are greater than this, but by how much depends on the type of epilepsy that you have. Some very rare epilepsies can be inherited by up to 50 per cent of children. Of the common epilepsies, the idiopathic generalized epilepsies (childhood absence, juvenile myoclonic epilepsy) have a higher risk of about 15–20 per cent for any child. However, these are mild epilepsies, the risk of which should not affect the decision to have a family. For most people with epilepsy, the risk of children developing the condition is little different from the population as a whole. If you do have concerns, discuss if first with your epilepsy specialist, who can, if necessary, refer you to specialist genetic services.

What are the risks of taking anti-epileptic medication during pregnancy?
Most people agree that it is best to avoid any drug, including both alcohol and tobacco, during pregnancy. However, a woman with active epilepsy will still need to continue anti-epileptic medication as the dangers of not taking medication and running the risk of having a seizure are generally greater than the risk associated with taking anti-epileptic drugs. The risk for the general population of having a child with a physical abnormality is about 2–3 per cent. The risk to the child of a woman on anti-epileptic medication is two to three times as great. Some of this increased risk is due to anti-epileptic medication taken throughout the pregnancy. If two or more anti-epileptic drugs are taken in combination the risk rises and it may rise further if large doses of the medication are being taken. Phenytoin, phenobarbitone and possibly

sodium valproate and carbamazepine have been associated with specific abnormalities. Phenytoin and phenobarbitone are associated with hare lip and cleft palate and sometimes with malformations of the heart. Fortunately, when these do occur they may often be corrected by operation.

Sodium valproate and carbamazepine may be associated with children being born with neural tube defects or spina bifida.

Medication

It is very important for all women with epilepsy to talk to the doctor responsible for their epilepsy treatment *before conception* or, if not, as early on in pregnancy as possible. If they have been free of seizures for more than two or three years the doctor may think about withdrawing anti-epileptic medication. The possible effect of having a further seizure on the woman's lifestyle, i.e. losing her driving licence, must be considered. If she is still having seizures, the doctor will wish to make sure that she is on the lowest dose of the most effective treatment which gives best control of her seizures. Any changes to medication should *always* be under the supervision of the doctor. We would now recommend that any woman taking anti epileptic drugs who is considering pregnancy should take folic acid supplements. This is a vitamin which has been shown to reduce the risks of a range of problems with pregnancy. Indeed, as many pregnancies are unplanned, it is sensible to take these vitamin supplements if you are sexually active. Your doctor can prescribe them.

During a pregnancy, the body uses up more of the anti-epileptic medication and the levels of the drug within the blood may fall, so blood levels should be monitored regularly and the dose adjusted accordingly.

Pregnancy should not present any special problems, although it is impossible to predict what will happen to each person. Some women do have seizures more frequently during pregnancy, but an equal number have them less frequently. The majority of women with epilepsy experience no major change.

Seizures during pregnancy

Will I have an increase in seizures during pregnancy?
The majority of women with epilepsy do not have an increased number of seizures during pregnancy but where this happens (in approximately a quarter of women) the increase is often due to anti-epileptic medication not being taken as prescribed, or not working properly because of vomiting, sleep deprivation or because being pregnant sometimes causes drug levels in the blood to fall. Epilepsy is better controlled during pregnancy in about half of all women and this is often because they are more careful about getting enough sleep, eating well and taking their medication regularly.

Seizures during labour

Only a very few women (1–2 per cent) with active epilepsy will have a seizure in labour and a further 1–2 per cent will have one in the next 24 hours. The general advice is to have your baby in hospital where doctors and midwives will do all they can to ensure that you are well looked after and that your baby's arrival is safe and happy. It is important to remember the following points:

● Make sure that you take your anti-epileptic medication during labour. Ask your partner or a nurse to keep a check on this for you in case you forget.
● Tell the midwife and the other staff on the ward about your epilepsy and the times at which you have to take your medication.
● Explain what form your seizures take and how they can help you if one occurs.

Remember that most women with epilepsy have perfectly normal deliveries.

Child care

Breast feeding

Breast feeding is to be encouraged and in women with epilepsy this is no exception. Even if the woman with epilepsy is taking anti-epileptic medication, breast feeding is not affected, as the baby has already been exposed to the drugs whilst in the womb. A problem that may arise with breast feeding, however, is sleep disturbance. If being short of sleep makes your seizures more likely, a partner, using a bottle, may help with some of the night-time feeds.

A good precaution against the risk of dropping the baby during a seizure is for the mother to sit on floor cushions and lean against the wall whilst breast feeding.

Looking after your baby

If your seizures are well controlled, the fact that you have epilepsy will not greatly interfere with looking after your child. In cases where your seizures are not well controlled, then certain risks do exist which will depend on the nature of your seizures. If seizures are sudden and unpredictable, dressing, changing, feeding and bathing the child should be carried out on the floor. If you are by yourself the baby should not be bathed in deep water and sponging the baby down on a changing mat on the floor is a safer alternative. Mothercare sell changing mats which are ideal for this purpose. Do not place the mat on a bed or table from which the child may fall.

Once your baby is mobile, it is important to make sure that fires, electrical appliances and other potential dangers are adequately guarded. You may consider using a play pen; this may help reduce the risk to a baby once it is mobile.

Looking after babies and small children can create problems, but none of these need be insurmountable, as can be seen from Sue Usiskin's story. Further recommendations about safety in the home will be found in the next chapter.

What about immunization?

Department of Health guidelines about immunization are

given in their publication *Immunisation against Infectious Disease*. The most recent edition was written in 1992. The whooping cough vaccine is generally the one which causes greatest concern. Here the Department of Health guidelines state that where there is a personal or family history of febrile convulsions immunization is recommended, with advice being given on preventing fever should this occur after being immunized. Similarly, if there is a family history of epilepsy, immunization is generally recommended.

The guidelines also state that:

No child should be denied immunisation without serious thought as to the consequences, both for the individual child and for the community. Where there is doubt advice should be sought from a Consultant Paediatrician, Consultant in Public Health Medicine or District [Health Board] Immunisation Co-ordinator.

The middle years

The menopause

In recent years women's health has gained more medical attention. A stage that has received particular attention for a number of good reasons is the menopause.

The average age for this change, when the menstrual periods stop and a woman can no longer become pregnant, is about 51. Most women notice changes in their cycle at any time in their 40s when they may experience hot flushes and rapid changes of mood. Some of the other unpleasant characteristics which may be associated with the menopause may be psychological or occur only occasionally.

The menopause often coincides with grown up children leaving home for the first time or a partner's retirement and also aged parents in declining health. Efforts should be made to develop new interests and to maintain existing ones. This will help you keep in good physical and psychological health. Hormone replacement therapy (HRT) may be recommended to relieve some of the more trying physical symptoms if they occur. There are many different types of hormone treatment available and these should be discussed with your doctor. An oestrogen supplement may be prescribed to prevent you losing too much calcium from your bones, a process known as osteoporosis. If bones become increasingly thin and brittle there is a danger that they will break more easily.

Very little research has been done on the effect of hormone treatment and epilepsy, so it is advisable to take each case on its merits. If your doctor strongly recommends HRT to protect your bones and also the heart, then epilepsy should not be seen as any form of contraindication. Epilepsy can also develop at any stage of life and some women will develop it at this time purely coincidentally.

It may be difficult to accept epilepsy at this time of life which, for some women, can present enough problems without additional complications. Good medical care and clear information are important so that you may experience the minimum of discomfort during this time; these should be available from your GP and the local Well Woman Clinic or Family Planning Clinic. Your GP should be able to recommend the best facility for you in your area.

You may be relieved to know that the physical and emotional changes experienced during middle age – notably the menopause – should not make any difference to your epilepsy.

Elderly people

One disease of later years that may produce epilepsy is stroke (*see page 42*). An elderly relative with epilepsy can be a special worry, particularly as the condition can arise in people who are handicapped by strokes or suffering senile dementia. With an elderly person who has these complicated disabilities, a degree of patience and understanding is essential.

Drug treatment is nearly always successful in stopping seizures. However, the elderly are particularly sensitive to the side-effects of anti-epileptic drugs, which can cause unsteadiness, drowsiness and confusion, often because they have to take a number of other drugs at the same time. Talk to your doctor if this seems to have reached an unacceptable level. An adjustment in your relative's medication should be possible.

Is special nursing necessary?
Epilepsy is rarely such a major problem in old age. If a relative does become too ill or difficult to look after at home, this will probably be due to a combination of problems and your decision as to the best care will have to be taken after discussion with your doctor and the rest of the family.

Psychological issues

Having epilepsy may cause difficulties in some areas of your life and may affect how you feel. People respond in different ways and some become angry, blaming themselves or life in general for what has happened to them. At first, many are confused, afraid and uncertain. These feelings may affect their ability to cope with daily activities, relationships with friends and family, and their self-esteem. They may have all sorts of misconceptions about their condition and imagine things to be worse than they are. Their need for emotional support and understanding from those around them increases and yet some may behave in a manner which seems rejecting.

Denial is a common response to any unpleasant news, but to adjust successfully to epilepsy you must first accept that you have it. The element of uncertainty that has crept into your life must not become the excuse for getting you out of everything. Seizures are not the only thing in life about which we have not had a choice; there are many other things we know we cannot change and have had to adapt to.

In order to live successfully with epilepsy it is important to learn a little about the disorder.

Basic knowledge

Knowing the facts about epilepsy and understanding and how they apply to you is essential. It is up to you to find out as much as you can about your condition and how you can look after yourself. This will diminish many stresses and anxieties to help you feel in control of your life rather than it controlling you! The way you think about epilepsy can do much to change your life. The following is a check list to help you gain a basic knowledge of your condition:

Diagnosis
- Do you know your type of epilepsy and its cause?
- What are your seizures like and what are they called?

Medication
- Do you know the name of your medication and the purpose of it?
- Do you understand the importance of taking medicines regularly?
- Do you know the common side effects of the drugs you are taking?
- Do you know about any possible interactions with the oral contraceptive?
- Do you know what to do if you miss a dose or vomit?
- Do you know that medicines for epilepsy are exempt from prescription charges?

Information
- Do you know where to find information on epilepsy?
- Have all your questions been answered?

Work

Employment benefits both self-esteem and social skills. A wide variety of jobs is open to people with epilepsy. Whether you are suited to a particular job depends both on your own talents and on the nature of your epilepsy. Indeed, your talents, qualifications and experience should be fully considered in relation to the job on offer before the effect of your epilepsy.

People with very infrequent seizures or seizures that occur only at particular times of the day – such as during sleep or first thing in the morning – will find there are few jobs for which they cannot be considered. People with more severe epilepsy and frequent, unpredictable seizures probably have a more limited scope.

How do you find a job?
The first step is to look at the same sources as everyone else – Job Centres, newspaper advertisements and employment

agencies, and for school and college leavers, the careers advisory service.

There are also special sources of advice: for school leavers, the specialist careers officer; at a Job Centre, people with epilepsy may request the help of the disability employment advisor (DEA), who has special responsibility for people with a variety of disabilities. The DEA may be able to direct you to a specialized training scheme that will provide useful experience and training. Finally, the Employment Medical Advisory Service (EMAS) provides advice to people looking for work as well as to employers about jobs that may be suitable.

A big difficulty is knowing how much information to give to a prospective employer, and when. It is certainly necessary to say that you have or have had epilepsy, unless it was a very long time ago. Not doing so could lead to dismissal without any protection under the Employment Acts. Ideally, you should not have to declare you have epilepsy on an initial application form. The Civil Service is an ideal employer in this respect: it does not ask for medical information on the first application form, but only after the job has been offered. Your medical suitability is then decided by a doctor who is a specialist in occupational health. Unfortunately, not all employers have such good practices. Too often the declaration of epilepsy can lead to an application being rejected by someone who has little or no understanding of the condition. It is usually best to leave blank those parts of a first application form that require medical information. However, if you do this you must declare your epilepsy if you are offered employment.

Which jobs are unsuitable?
1. If you have had even a single epileptic seizure it will be difficult to work driving heavy goods or public service vehicles or taxis. You would now be required to go for at least 10 years without seizures *and* 10 years without taking anti-epileptic drugs before being allowed this type of licence. You are unlikely ever to be allowed a pilot's licence or to become a train driver.
2. You should be careful about trying for jobs where you need

to drive at all, as further seizures can lead to your losing your licence *(see page 97)*.

3. Avoid jobs that involve working at heights.
4. If you have frequent seizures, you should avoid factory work and working with heavy machinery, although this sort of work should be possible if you have a less severe form of epilepsy. Any machinery must be adequately guarded, regardless of whether workers have epilepsy.
5. You will find it difficult to gain admission to schools of nursing and medicine. Individual schools follow different rules, and each case is considered on its merits, but people with active epilepsy will not be able to practise surgery or anaesthesia.
6. A history of epilepsy will prevent admission to the armed services, police and fire services.
7. People in the armed services who develop epilepsy will usually be downgraded medically, which reduces their prospects of promotion.
8. You can teach most subjects if you have epilepsy, but there may be restrictions placed on teaching physical education and other subjects such as chemistry.
9. If your epilepsy is not completely controlled you may have problems gaining work with young children or near open water.

Although the Disabled Persons (Employment) Act of 1944 provides that employers with 20 or more employees have a duty to employ disabled people to fill at least 3 per cent of their workforce, it has never been enforced legally, so no one has to employ a person with epilepsy. You have to show yourself to have the appropriate talents and qualifications and be willing to sell yourself in an interview. You may have to work harder to get the job you want than people without your condition. You are not alone. Other groups of people with different disadvantages have to overcome them too. Persistence pays off in the end. Try to resist the temptation to blame epilepsy for any failures – the explanation may be something quite simple, like high unemployment with many people applying for the same job.

Unemployment

A period of unemployment may be unavoidable these days. Not everybody is able to find a suitable job when they want one and as inactivity and boredom may increase the likelihood of seizures, you should try to avoid this.

A period of voluntary work or a college course will show a future employer that you are keen and interested in acquiring new skills. It will also provide you with a routine, regular hours and better social skills. Ideas about local voluntary work schemes can be found from the Citizen's Advice Bureaux and Community Volunteers.

Unemployment and other benefits do change, so for more information check with your local Social Services or the Benefits Enquiry Line (BEL), England, Scotland and Wales telephone 0800 882 200, and Northern Ireland telephone 0800 220 674 during working hours. Staff give advice and offer a claims completion form service.

Pensions, trade unions and insurance

There should not be a problem with any one of these provided that you are open about the facts. Some people say that these requirements present problems which prevent them from employing people with epilepsy. You can dispel these ideas by knowing that:

- No special insurance is necessary for a worker with epilepsy. The employer's liability insurance covers everyone in the workplace on the understanding that in allocating work the employer takes account of the nature of the individual's disability.
- It is the policy of the Occupational Pensions Board that if someone is fit enough to be an employee, they are acceptable for a pension scheme if one exists.
- Machinery must be adequately guarded in order to comply with the safety regulations protecting all workers; this should prevent injury should a seizure happen, but if special guards are required, subsidies are obtainable from the Employment Service (via the DEA).

- The TUC and virtually all trade unions have positive policies on the employment of people with disabilities; where there are allegations of discrimination at work because of epilepsy, the trade union should be able to help.

A positive approach

About 100,000 people with epilepsy work in the UK today. Research has shown that on average, they have fewer accidents than the other employees. They also take less time off work and have good job loyalty records (as they value their jobs so highly!)

Remember that you must be adequately trained with the appropriate skills for the job that you are applying for in order to stand a good chance of being employed. At interview, be prepared to explain clearly any facts which may make your condition more understandable to a prospective employer. The Epilepsy Association publish some useful information leaflets to help you with this, such as *Explaining Epilepsy* and *Seizures*. Practising explaining about your epilepsy may be helpful before the interview and practice in front of a mirror or with a friend or family member may help you to gain the confidence you need.

Leisure

The amount of time people have for leisure is steadily increasing. A full and active life is important for everyone and there is no need to be over-restrictive when making your choices as to which activity to pursue. Common sense should be the main factor in deciding which activities you can take up and provided that you take the same safety precautions as everyone else you should come to no harm.

Choosing an activity

If your epilepsy is fully controlled by anti-epileptic medication this will be more straightforward. If not, in deciding whether or not to take part in an activity you should ask yourself, 'Is this realistic and safe, given my seizure type?'

Children with epilepsy at school should be included in the full range of sport as far as possible, provided sensible precautions are taken.

The following advice may help you adopt sensible safety measures and help minimize potential risks:

- **Ball games:** There is no reason why most people with epilepsy but no other physical disabilities should not play football, rugby, cricket, rounders or netball.
- **Climbing:** Never climb alone. If your epilepsy is well controlled and you are a keen climber, it is important to climb only when safety ropes are used in an organized group and with a professional guide. Be sure that the guide knows you have epilepsy and how to help you should you have a seizure, and that they are happy to take this responsibility. Climbing trees is a popular activity with children. Try to make the dangers clear to your child and to restrict climbing to safe sites.
- **Cycling:** If you have frequent seizures, avoid cycling on busy roads. It is advisable to cycle with a friend or in a group. Cycling helmets are recommended for everyone.
- **Discos and nightclubs:** These are an important part of the social life of many young people. Again, those with photosensitive epilepsy may find that they can have seizures triggered by strobe (flashing) lights, though the frequency of flash makes this unusual.
- **Riding:** As for cycling, hard hats should be worn by anyone riding and if your epilepsy is not well controlled you are advised to ride with someone who would know what to do in the event of a seizure. The organization Riding for the Disabled provides local groups where activities are supervised *(see Useful Addresses section at the end of the book)*.
- **Swimming:** It is advisable when swimming to be accompanied by a strong swimmer who knows you have epilepsy and could come to your aid if you were to have an attack in the water. A lifeguard at the pool should be informed about the possibility of seizures and what form they take. Watersports such as sailing, canoeing and windsurfing must be regarded as carrying a greater degree

of risk and more dangerous watersports such as sub-aqua diving, which involve much greater risks, are not advised.

- **Television and computer games:** If you are unsure as to whether or not your epilepsy is photosensitive, your doctor will advise you. Do not sit too near to the screen and take regular breaks away from it. Change channels on the TV using a remote control rather than going too close to the screen.
- **Yoga:** Many people find that yoga is beneficial. The deep breathing involved in many forms of yoga is unlikely to cause difficulties and may be very relaxing. National yoga associations may provide further information.

Computer games

There has been a lot of publicity about epilepsy and computer games. The facts need to be clearly understood as the chances of a seizure being triggered are in fact very small.

It is known that flashing lights and certain strong geometric patterns such as stripes are some of the environmental triggers which occasionally precipitate seizures. Fortunately only a small proportion (3 per cent) of people with epilepsy will have the potential to have seizures induced by flashing lights or geometric patterns and this is more common in children than in adults. The risks of seizures can be reduced by the precautions described *(see page 39)*.

Special holiday schemes

There are some publications available which list organizations providing holidays for people with epilepsy as well as those with other disabilities. The Royal Association for Disability and Rehabilitation (RADAR) produces *Holidays and Travel Abroad* and *Holidays in the British Isles*. The organization PHAB runs clubs, holidays and schemes around the UK which bring physically disabled and able bodied people together *(see Useful Addresses section)*.

Support groups – are they helpful?

The British Epilepsy Association and National Society for Epilepsy organize a number of regional support groups for people with epilepsy and their families. They can be unrepresentative of the general population with epilepsy as they often have a lot of people with very severe epilepsy attending. If you have been recently diagnosed you may find this rather frightening and should be aware of it before deciding whether or not a support group is for you. There may also be some people with special needs attending who have other disabilities besides epilepsy.

Groups vary enormously in their size and what they offer. Some groups have active education programmes with invited speakers and others are organized purely on a social basis. Support groups can be a positive help and benefit for those who feel particularly isolated by their diagnosis. They may offer an opportunity for you to meet others with epilepsy living in your area and to learn more about the condition.

More able people with epilepsy can be a great help to those who are more severely affected. If your condition is relatively mild, you may feel inclined to help in this way. Support groups are organized by the major national epilepsy charities *(see Useful Addresses)*. If there is no epilepsy support group in your area and you wish to start one up, contact one of the epilepsy charities for help and advice.

Alcohol

Alcohol plays a role in many social activities, and you need to treat it with particular respect for two reasons:

1. The drugs that are used to treat epilepsy do not mix well with alcohol. They can make the effects of alcohol more marked.
2. Alcohol can make seizures more likely. You may well have a seizure a day or two after a bout of heavy drinking.

While it is not necessary to be teetotal, you should have no more than one or two alcoholic drinks during the course of an evening. Sometimes the labels on bottles of drugs used to treat epilepsy state that the medication should not be taken with alcohol. As a result people sometimes make the mistake of not taking their drugs because they know they are going to have a drink. That is, of course, the worst of all possible situations; you must take your medication regularly.

Travel

Careful planning can make travel enjoyable and whether you are going at home or abroad the following precautions may enhance your enjoyment:

- Make sure you have enough medication to last you through your trip and if you are travelling by air, always travel with spare medication in your hand luggage, in case your baggage is delayed or lost.
- Take a copy of your prescription to prove you need medication for a medical condition and for replacement purposes. (In some countries your drugs may be illegal – if you are concerned you may check with the consultant before travelling.)
- *The Traveller's Handbook for People with Epilepsy* gives helpful suggestions and is available from the following address with a stamped, self-addressed envelope: IBE, PO Box 21, 2100 A A Heemstede, The Netherlands.
- If you have frequent seizures and are flying for the first time, you may wish to tell the cabin stewards about your epilepsy and how to help you during an attack. Flying itself will not cause seizures, but international travel may disturb regular sleeping times. If you are travelling a long way, try to plan flights that will lead to the least possible disturbance to your sleep.
- Make sure you have adequate medical insurance before you travel.
- Medical facilities are available and you can afford them. Medical expenses which are incurred in EU countries may be reclaimed by completing form E111 before you travel.

Driving

This is part of everyday life for many people, but the laws that govern the right of people with epilepsy to drive are strict. Neither your own doctor nor the doctors in the medical department of the Driver and Vehicle Licensing Agency (DVLA) have any great discretion in the way that these rules are applied.

If you have epilepsy or have had a single seizure, you will not be allowed to hold an ordinary driving licence until 12 months have gone by without any seizures. This means that even if you are having only relatively minor auras, you may not drive a car or motorcycle. The one exception to this rule is that people whose fits occur only during sleep may hold a driving licence if they have had fits only during sleep for a period of at least three years.

The rules about Group II licences (the old heavy goods and public service vehicle licences) are more strict and demand 10 years without seizures *and* at least 10 years off all anti-epileptic drugs before a licence can be granted.

When you have been diagnosed as having epilepsy, your doctor will tell you about these regulations and explain how they apply to you, but it is your responsibility to inform the licensing authorities. The driving licence states that you must inform the DVLA at once if you have any disability that is or may become likely to affect your fitness as a driver. You should not drive in the period between informing the DVLA and receiving a reply.

After you have gone for 12 months without any attacks, you can apply for a driving licence. The DVLA will obtain information from your own doctor and almost certainly accept your application. Your licence will be reviewed at three-yearly intervals until seven years after your last seizure, when you will be given an 'until 70 licence'.

It is vital that everyone observes these regulations, for the risks are very real. Unfortunately, some people still ignore the law. In a survey of 2,000 road accidents that were due to the driver collapsing at the wheel, 50 per cent were caused by epilepsy. Of those caused by epilepsy, 70 per cent of the drivers had a previous history of the condition and had failed to inform the DVLA.

Insurance

If you continue to drive after the diagnosis of epilepsy, not only are you doing so without a valid licence, but also without insurance cover. You must inform your insurance company of your epilepsy when you get your licence, or get it reinstated, or they may refuse to cover you for any liabilities.

Safety in the home

Most people with epilepsy can live independently perfectly safely. There are, however, a number of precautions you should always observe, whatever type of epilepsy you have, to guard against accidents during an unexpected seizure.

Alarms

A variety of alarm systems has been developed and these range from the simplest to the more sophisticated. If your seizures are frequent and involve falling, you might be helped by one of the following:

- Fallcall is a system that activates an alarm when the wearer falls. It also alerts people to a card which the wearer carries and which has instructions about what to do to help. Clip-on or pendant models are available and the design is robust. The unit is neat and several different models are available. For further information contact: Fallcall Systems Limited, 5 Park Lane, Barnstaple, North Devon, EX32 9AJ; telephone (01271) 44426.
- Bed alarms are available from Aremco, Grove House, Lenham, Kent, ME17 2PX; telephone (01622) 858502.

Bathing

Care needs to be taken when bathing, especially by people whose epilepsy is not well controlled. It is a good idea to let someone know that you are going to take a bath before getting in. A shower may be preferable to a bath and showers with high-sided bases should be avoided since they may trap water if you were to fall and cover the drain.

It is safer not to lock the door. An 'engaged' sign on an unlocked door allows privacy but means that someone can get to you if necessary. An 'engaged' sign on an unlocked toilet door may also be useful.

Beds and pillows

If you have night-time seizures, placing the bed against the wall and using floor cushions around it to prevent injury may help. A low level bed or futon gives added protection. Avoid smoking in bed, as this could result in a fire. Special safety pillows which reduce the risk of suffocation are available from Helpful Hands, 2 Chester Road, Macclesfield, Cheshire, SK10 1AU; telephone (01625) 617857, though for the majority of people with epilepsy this precaution will not be necessary.

DIY

If your epilepsy is not well controlled, avoid climbing high ladders. Electric saws and screwdrivers should not be used when you are alone.

Doors

Safety glass in doors and low windows minimizes risk of injury if your seizures involve falling. Alternatively, glass safety film is available from Mothercare and, if applied to glass, helps prevent splintering.

Bathroom and toilet doors may be hung so that they open outwards. This prevents the door becoming blocked by a person falling behind it. If using locks, use safety locks which can be operated from outside.

Electric sockets

An adequate number of sockets prevents trailing flexes, which can be very dangerous if appliances are pulled over.

First aid

A fully stocked first-aid kit is useful for treating minor injuries.

Furniture

Avoid injury from falling against furniture with sharp corners by fitting plastic corner covers (available from Mothercare). If you are a smoker, fireproof fabrics and furniture are more widely available now and should be considered.

Kitchen equipment

Reduce injuries by using microwave ovens and the special plastic microwaveable containers instead of glass dishes. When using a conventional cooker, use the back rings or burners rather than those at the front. Turn the saucepan handles away from the edge and grill food rather than frying it, or use the oven and close the door.

Other things to consider are:

- cordless irons (without trailing flexes)
- automatic cordless jug kettles with safety lids and safety cutout
- cooker guards (available from Mothercare)
- a trolley to transfer food and hot dishes from the oven to the table

Heating

Avoid light free-standing heaters which can be easily knocked over if you fall. Fire guards should be firmly secured for open or metal cased fires. Radiator guards are an added precaution.

Medication

Take care with your medication and how you store it, particularly if you have young children about. Your anti-epileptic and any other drugs must be locked away. Should you need to carry them with you, avoid carrying more than you need for that day.

Safety outside the home

It may be a good idea to carry or wear something which says you have epilepsy. Bracelets and necklaces are available from the Medic-Alert Foundation, 12 Bridge Wharf, 156 Caledonian Road, London N1 9UU; telephone 0171–833 3034; and also SOS Talisman, Talman Ltd, 21 Grays Court, Ley Street, Ilford, Essex, IG2 7RQ; telephone 0181–554 5579.

The National Society for Epilepsy produce a free information card which can be carried in a plastic wallet. The card can hold personal details, information on what type of seizures you have, what treatment you are on and information on how to manage seizures. These are available from the Information Dept., The National Society for Epilepsy, Chalfont St. Peter, Gerrards Cross, Bucks, SL9 ORJ. Please enclose an SAE.

Stairs

If your seizures are frequent or unpredictable, stairs may be dangerous. Careful planning may keep the number of occasions that you use the stairs to a minimum.

Further help

Further help is available from all epilepsy associations *(see Useful Addresses at the back of the book)*.

Acceptance

The fact that you have bought this book and are reading it is a sign that you have accepted that you have epilepsy. An important part of the journey towards acceptance involves your doctor and the relationship you are able to have with him or her. People vary greatly in what they know. An experienced doctor, specialist nurse or counsellor will certainly have come across every possible kind of question from patients and will not be surprised by anything that you ask.

Sometimes it is helpful to make a list of questions you want to discuss to take along with you to an appointment. In some cases you may find that your doctor cannot say what has caused your epilepsy and you may feel that this makes it harder for you to accept the condition. Remember that doctors are limited by the current knowledge available and, like other professionals, they can only do their best. Anyone can develop epilepsy and, despite what was thought centuries ago, epilepsy is not a punishment for bad behaviour. If you are able to make full use of the positive aspects of your life it will help you a great deal to see epilepsy in perspective.

Remember epilepsy can be satisfactorily controlled in about 80 per cent of cases with medication taken regularly. It does not usually grow worse with age and often improves after a period of time. The majority of people with epilepsy are of normal intelligence and able to lead full lives. Do not be a helpless victim – there are things that you can do!

Anxiety

One of the psychological consequences of living with epilepsy is a certain level of anxiety. Seizures may be frequent or infrequent, they may happen in public during the daytime or at night when you are alone. Uncertainty about when and if the next attack will occur presents a particular problem. You may be living with an ever-present threat, never knowing when the next seizure will happen. People who do not have epilepsy usually think that the person with epilepsy is 'normal' between seizures. You may not agree! On the other hand, it is fruitless to sacrifice your entire life if at every moment you are thinking you might have a seizure. In fact, seizures only take up a very small percentage of your life and it is important to make the most of all the rest of the time when you are not having one. Sometimes, the reaction of people to you when you have a seizure will be upsetting and may cause you to feel anxious. Try to remember that people do not respond to everything the way one would like and that the world is far from perfect. Often people just do not understand what they are seeing and do not know how to help. This is one of the main reasons why some people pass by or do nothing. Other people do the wrong thing and may cause you some damage accidentally. It is hard to remember that was not their intention, they simply did not know any better. Another reason why some people may ignore you is embarrassment. They may feel uncomfortable about their ignorance and feel embarrassed about it.

The more open you can be about your epilepsy, the more people will feel at ease with you and able to ask you questions about it. Sometimes it may feel to you as if no one wants to know about your condition, but they may be picking up on a feeling that you do not really feel comfortable talking about it. All this promotes anxiety and only you gradually have the power to change things.

Relaxation

If you are inclined to be anxious, learning how to relax will be important. How you do this is largely a matter of choice. Try to allocate specific times in your routine for relaxation. Some people find that yoga, with its emphasis on deep breathing, is helpful. Dancing is a means of relaxation and self-expression and if you enjoy music, dancing may be the perfect way to relax either alone or with friends.

Walking can be very relaxing and good exercise. A brisk walk in attractive surroundings can be enjoyable whatever the weather, providing that you are suitably dressed. While you are out walking you may enjoy listening to music or book tapes on a personal stereo.

Some complementary therapies such as aromatherapy, reflexology and acupuncture are sources of relaxation to some people and the best thing is to try them out and see which one you like. Do not expect them to cure your epilepsy; the reason for pursuing them is for relaxation and enjoyment. You can buy relaxation tapes which are specially designed to help you become more aware of the areas of tension in your body and which suggest ways of dealing with this, such as concentrating the mind and breathing exercises.

Advice about swimming and other sport is given under Leisure *(see page 93)*.

Section III

Managing Epilepsy

7

Treatment

Epileptic fits can be dramatic and frightening events. People seeing one for the first time feel an understandable desire to interfere and to try to protect the person having the attack. It is important to remember that seizures are self-limiting and that, in the vast majority of cases, people are not seriously injured. The list on page 22 explains what you should and should not do to help someone having a seizure.

Most people who have epilepsy need to take drugs to prevent further attacks. The success of your treatment depends on your taking medication regularly; forgetting to do this is perhaps the commonest reason for treatment failing. Many people do not have any further attacks after they start the treatment.

When to start anti-epileptic drugs

In the past people were sometimes given anti-epileptic drugs even before they had a seizure. People who suffer very severe head injuries or who have particular kinds of neurosurgical operations do have a high risk of developing epilepsy and so at one time neurosurgeons gave them anti-epileptic drugs. However, there is little evidence that starting treatment at this stage prevents the development of epilepsy and it meant that many people were receiving unnecessary medication.

We know that having one seizure does not mean that someone has epilepsy. As many as 70 per cent of people who have not had a second attack within six to eight weeks of their first will never have another. For this reason it is now usual not to treat people until they have had at least two epileptic seizures. Even some people who have had two seizures will not need treatment. Each case needs very careful considera-tion. Most doctors probably would not start treatment if a person's attacks were' very infrequent, perhaps less than one every one to two years. Some people who have had more frequent attacks might not need treatment if a clear provoking factor can be identified. For example, children with febrile convulsions *(see page 36)*, or people who have fits provoked only by flashing lights or by alcohol withdrawal usually do not need treatment; they and their families simply need advice about avoiding the provoking factors.

A person's attitude towards treatment is important and if you feel any reluctance about accepting it you should discuss this frankly with your doctor.

Starting anti-epileptic treatment

Problem	Usual clinical practice	Modifying factors
Prospective risk of epilepsy	No treatment	
Single isolated seizure	No treatment	Progressive cerebral disorder. Clearly abnormal EEG.
Two or more	Monotherapy	Seizures more than one year apart. Identified precipitating factors (drugs, alcohol, photic stimuli) Patient acceptance.

Choosing the right drug

The aim is always to control epilepsy with the simplest possible drug regime that has the fewest side-effects. Therefore it is usual to begin treatment with a small dose of a single drug. In many cases this stops attacks; the dose will be increased gradually only if you have further attacks. Your doctor will decide which drug to give you after very careful consideration of the following:

1. Which drugs are likely to be most effective against the kind of epilepsy you have?
2. Which of the effective drugs is likely to have the fewest side-effects?
3. Which of the effective drugs will be easiest for you to take?

The drugs used to treat epilepsy, the kinds of epilepsy for which they are used and their more common side-effects are summarized in the table on pages 112–116.

Payment for drugs and further assistance

In the UK people with epilepsy are exempt from prescription charges for anti-epileptic drugs. You should get leaflet P11 from the post office, fill in form C and send it to your doctor to sign. If your fits are so frequent that you need attendance during the day and night, you might be able to obtain a disability living allowance. Information and instructions on how to claim can be obtained from your social security office.

There are a number of epilepsy associations which provide information, advice and social contacts for people with epilepsy and raise money for research (*see Useful Addresses section*).

Names of drugs

Many drugs have at least two names. The chemical, or generic, name is given first in the table and the text, and the proprietary, or trade, name is given second. For example, phenytoin is the generic name of the drug that is sold as Epanutin by the manufacturer Parke-Davis. A pharmacist might provide either the generic or the proprietary drug when a prescription is made out for the generic, so you might be given either phenytoin or Epanutin if your doctor has prescribed phenytoin. In the case of phenytoin it is important that people are not changed from the generic to the propriet-ary drug or vice versa, as differing amounts of the drug pass into the body from the two formulations. The difference between generic and proprietary versions of other drugs is not so crucial.

Indications

This tells you for which kinds of epilepsy a drug is used. Usage is described in the table on pages 112–116 in three ways:

1. Drug of choice: also called a 'first line' drug; that is, the preferred one.
2. Effective drug: a 'second line' drug, used when the drug of choice is not available or not satisfactory.
3. Occasional use: a drug that might be used, but usually only when the first and second line drugs have proved unsatisfactory.

Side-Effects

Drugs can produce side-effects, and these are categorized in the table as follows:

- **Dose related:** Effects that anyone can have, given high enough doses, but which will disappear when the dose is reduced.
- **Allergic:** Reactions that occur rarely, unpredictably and usually soon after the drug is started, and will recur if it is taken again; many reactions such as rashes are true allergies, but the ways that others develop are less certain.
- **Chronic toxicity:** Effects that develop slowly, after prolonged use. These are more common in people taking large doses of more than one drug.

The commonest dose-related side-effect is intoxication, or 'drunkenness'. Particularly with phenobarbitone, phenytoin, primidone, carbamazepine and lamotrigine, this can cause dizziness, difficulty with concentration, unsteadiness in walking, slurred speech and double vision.

Older drugs tend to have more side-effects than those introduced more recently. For example, many people who take phenobarbitone, and to a lesser degree phenytoin, even in moderate doses, feel rather tired, sleepy and sedated, and we can measure the adverse effect on memory, alertness and reaction time. The newer drugs carbamazepine and valproate have fewer effects of this nature and have become first choice drugs. Phenobarbitone, primidone and phenytoin can have unpleasant cosmetic effects, causing acne and facial hairiness, which are unpleasant for women. Phenytoin can also be difficult to use because even quite small increases in the dose can cause a large rise in its concentration in the blood, and symptoms of intoxication. Frequent blood tests are usually necessary to check the concentration of phenytoin, whereas this is not necessary with carbamazepine and valproate.

Over recent years a number of new anti-epileptic drugs have been licensed in the United Kingdom and around the world. These are usually given at first to people with more severe epilepsy and we are only now beginning to be able to draw conclusions about how they compare with the older 'standard drugs'. These new drugs include vigabatrin (Sabril), lamotrigine (Lamictal), gabapentin (Neurontin), topiramate (Topamax) and tiagabine (Gabatril).

What should you do if you have side-effects?

If you develop 'drunkenness' you should go and see your own doctor, who will advise you about changing the drug dosage. It's not necessary to change the drug itself. These symptoms should settle within a few days of the change in your dose.

What should you do if you find it hard to remember your dose?

You certainly must tell your doctor if you are missing medication regularly. You may find it helpful to get one of the little boxes that can be divided up so that you can put the week's supply in. Then you can be sure you actually take your pills on the day and at the time when you should.

Optimal serum concentration

It is now possible to measure the concentration of a drug in a sample of blood. For many drugs we can define a range of levels below which there might be room for increased dosage and improved control of seizures, but above which there is an

Drug	Preparation	Interactions	Indications	Dosage	Optimal Serum concentration	Adverse effects
Generic name: Clobazam Trade name: Frisium Maker: Hoechst	10 mg tablets	Allosteric enhancement of GABA-mediated inhibition	Occasional use: tonic-clonic and partial seizures particularly perimenstrual; (value is limited by development of tolerance)	Adults: Up to 30 mg daily in 2 or 3 doses Children: >3 yr; half adult dose (maximum)	Not routinely measured	Dose-related: Drowsiness and sedation Allergic: — Chronic toxicity: —
Generic name: Carbamazepine Trade name: Tegretol Maker: Geigy	100, 200, 400 mg tablets 100mg/5ml syrup	Limits repetitive firing of Na+ dependent action potentials	Drug of choice: complex partial seizures (particularly if complicated by psychiatric disturbance), tonic-clonic, and simple partial seizures	Adults: 300–1,600 mg daily; initial dose low with slow increments (NB auto-induction of metabolism) Children: <1 yr 100–200 mg; 1–5 yr 200–400 mg; 5–10 yr 400–600 mg; 10–15 yr 0.6–1 g; or commence on 10mg/kg/day for 5–7 days; then 20–40 mg/kg/day thereafter	4–10 µg/ml (but little evidence to support this)	Dose related: Dizziness, double vision, unsteadiness, nausea, and vomiting Allergic: Rashes, reduced white cell count Chronic toxicity: Few known: absence of major effects on intellectual function and behavior is major benefit

| Generic name: **Clonazepam** Trade name: **Rivotril** Maker: **Roche** | 0.5, 2.0 mg tablets, 1 mg ampoules for intravenous injection. | Allosteric enhancement of GABA-mediated inhibition | Effective in: status epilepticus Effective in: absence, myoclonus Occasional use: slowly increasing doses tonic-clonic and partial seizures; (value greatly limited by development of tolerance) | **Adults:** Orally: 0.5–4 mg 3 times daily in slowly increasing doses **Children:** <1 yr 0.5–1 mg/day; 1–5 yr 1–3 mg/day; 6–12 yr 3–6 mg/day; *or* 0.1–0.2 mg/kg/day and usually commence on 0.02 mg/kg/day | Not routinely measured | **Dose-related:** Dizziness, double vision, unsteadiness, nausea, and vomiting **Allergic:** Inflammation of veins **Chronic toxicity:**— |
| Generic name: **Diazepam** Trade name: **Valium, Diazemuls, Stesolid** Maker: **Roche, KabiVitum, CP Pharmaceuticals** | **Valium** 2, 5, 10 mg tablets 2 mg/5ml syrup, 10ml ampoules tor I/V injection **Diazemuls** 10mg ampoules for I/V or rectal administration **Stesolid** 10 mg tubes for rectal administration | Allosteric enhancement of GABA-mediated inhibition | Effective in: status epilepticus, occasional use: absence, myoclonus; (value limited by development of tolerance) | **Adults:** Intravenous; rectal administration may be of value when venous access difficult; little effect orally; **Children:** 0.3–0.4 mg/kg (intravenous or rectal administration) | Not routinely measured | **Dose-related:** Sedation **Allergic:** — **Chronic toxicity:** Habituation |

Drug	Preparation	Interactions	Indications	Dosage	Optimal Serum concentration	Adverse effects
Generic name: Ethosuximaide Trade name: Zarontin, Emeside Maker: Parke-Davis, laboratories for applied medicine	250 mg capsules 250 mg / 5ml syrup	Reduce low-threshold calcium current	Drug of choice: simple absence	Adults: Up to 2 g / day in 2 or 3 doses Children: <6 yr 250 mg/day; >6 yr 0.5–1 g/day; or 20–40 mg/kg/day	40–80 µg/ml	Dose-related: Nausea drowsiness, dizziness, unsteadiness, may exacerbate tonic-clonic seizures Allergic: Rashes Chronic toxicity: Tolerance, habituation, withdrawal seizures; adverse effects on intellectual function and behavior
Generic name: Phenobarbitone Trade name: Gardenal, Luminal, Prominal Maker: May and Baker, Winthrop, SK and F	15 mg, 30 mg, 60 mg, 100 mg, 200 mg tablets 30 mg / 10 ml elixir, 60 mg, 100 mg, spansules	Enhancement of GABA-mediated inhibition	Effective in: tonic, clonic and partial seizures; occasional use: status epilepticus, absence, myoclonus	Adults: Up to 200 mg/day in 2 or 3 doses Children: Usually 4–5 mg/kg/day	15–35 µg/ml; upper and lower limits modified by development of tolerance	Dose-related: Drowsiness, unsteadiness Allergic Rashes Chronic-toxicity: Tolerance, habituation, withdrawal seizures; adverse effects on intellectual function and behavior
Generic name: Lamotrigine Trade name: Lamictal Maker: Wellcome	50 mg, 100 mg tablets 25 - 100 mg dispersable tablets	Has carbamazepine and phenytoin-like effect on repetitive firing	Refractory partial and secondary generalized seizures. Probably also effective in generalized epilepsy	Adults: 100–600 mg/ day; NB enzyme-inducing drugs reduce half-life, valproate increases it Children: —	1–3 µg/ml	Dose-related: Nausea and vomiting, headache, diplopia, aggression, swollen ankles Allergic: Rashes Chronic toxicity: Not yet known

Generic name / Trade name / Maker / Form	Mechanism	Effective in	Dose	Blood level	Side effects
Generic name: Phenytoin **Trade name:** Epanutin **Maker:** Parke-Davis — 25 mg, 50 mg, 100 mg capsules, 50 mg chewable tablets, 30 mg/5 ml suspension	Inhibits sustained repetitive firing effects on Na+-dependent voltage channels	Effective in: tonic-clonic, simple and complex partial seizures	**Adults:** 200–600 mg/day in 1 or 2 doses **Children:** 5–8 mg/kg/day	10–20 µg/ml; the non-linear relationship between dose and serum concentration necessitates frequent blood-level monitoring	**Dose-related:** Drowsiness, unsteadiness, slurred speech, occasionally abnormal movement disorders **Allergic:** Rashes, swelling of lymph glands (pseudolymphoma), hepatitis **Chronic toxicity:** Gingival hypertrophy, acne, coarsening of facial features, hirsutism, folate deficiency
Generic name: Primidone **Trade name:** Mysoline **Maker:** ICI — 250 mg tablets, 250 mg/ml suspension	As phenobarbitone	Occasional use: tonic-clonic and partial seizures	**Adults:** 500–1,500 mg/day in 2 or 3 doses **Children:** 10–30 mg/kg in 2 or 3 doses (rarely used)	As phenobarbitone—to whic it is metabolized	**Dose-related:** Drowsiness, unsteadiness, often tolerated poorly on initiation and a slow increase in dose advisable **Allergic:** See phenobarbitone **Chronic toxicity:** See phenobarbitone
Generic name: Sodium valproate **Trade name:** Epilim **Maker:** Merril Dow — 500 mg tablets	? Enhancement of GABA-mediated inhibition Limits sustained repetitive firing ? Reduces effects of excitatory neurotransmitters	Drug of choice: idiopathic generalized epilepsies, partial and secondary generalized seizures	**Adults:** 600–3,000 mg in 2 or 3 doses **Children:** 20–60 mg/kg/day (usually 20–30 mg/kg/day)	Uncertain: blood levels vary considerably during the day and a single specimen is unreliable	**Dose-related:** Tremor, irritability, restlessness; occasionally confusion **Allergic:** Gastric intolerance, hepatotoxicity (mainly children) **Chronic toxicity:** Weight gain: alopecia

Drug	Preparation	Interactions	Indications	Dosage	Optimal Serum concentration	Adverse effects
Generic name: **Vigabatrin** Trade name: **Sabril** Maker: **Parke-Davis**	100 mg, 300 mg, 400 mg capsules	Enzyme-activated suicidal inhibitor of GABA aminotransaminase	Treatment of partial epilepsy not satisfactorily controlled by other drugs	**Adults:** 2–4 g/day in 1 or 2 doses **Children:** 3–9 yr 1 g/day; >9 yr 2 g/day; or 50–150 mg/kg/day in 2 or 3 divided doses	Unrelated to known mode of action	**Dose-related:** Drowsiness and fatigue, nervousness, irritability, depression, confusion, altered memory, mild gastrointestinal disturbance **Allergic:** Psychosis **Chronic toxicity:** —
Generic name: **Gabapentin** Trade name: **Neurontin** Maker: **Parke-Davis**	100 mg, 300 mg, 400 mg capsules	May increase GABA release. Binds to unique receptor nature of which is uncertain	Refractory partial and secondarily generalized tonic-clonic seizures	**Adults:** 900–2,400 mg/day **Children:** No indication	—	**Dose-related:** Drowsiness, headache, tremor **Allergic:** None known **Chronic toxicity:** Not yet known
Generic name: **Topiramate** Trade name: **Topamax** Maker: **Janssen-Cilag**	25 mg, 100mg, 200mg tablets	Inactivates voltage-sensitive sodium channels. May bind to GABA receptors and have an action at glutaminergic receptors	Refractory partial and secondarily generalized tonic-clonic seizures	**Adults:** 200–800 mg/day **Children:** No indication	—	**Dose-related:** Impaired memory and cognition, drowsiness, paraesthesiae. **Allergic:** None known **Chronic toxicity:** Renal calculi, weight loss

increased risk of side-effects. Having this measurement taken can ensure that you are being given the correct dosage. This is important for drugs such as phenytoin but much less helpful for newer drugs.

Treatment for continuing seizures

A few people will continue to have seizures after they have started taking anti-epileptic drugs. They are most likely to be people who have partial seizures. What can be done in this situation? It is certainly reasonable to increase the dose of the original medication cautiously until either the attacks disappear or side-effects begin to develop. By having blood tests regularly to check the concentration of the drug, it is often possible to predict when side-effects might develop *(see page 110)*.

With increased doses of drugs, tonic-clonic seizures usually become less frequent and might stop, but sometimes it is difficult to prevent partial seizures taking place. Then the possibility of changing to another drug or of adding a second drug and having a trial period when you take a combination of drugs will have to be considered.

Doctors have, in the past, avoided combining drugs. Taking two, three or even four different ones can cause problems. They can interact with each other and you are certainly more likely to have side-effects if you take a combination. Each drug can on occasion interfere with the action of the others, so that it can be difficult to obtain satisfactory concentrations of drugs in the blood. Since there is no good evidence that people are better off on two drugs rather than one, let alone three rather than two, there is a powerful argument for keeping treatment simple and restricting it to a single drug whenever possible.

It is important to understand what expectations we can realistically have of drug treatment. Sometimes it can be extremely difficult to abolish a person's attacks completely and if your doctor has explained that this is true in your case, it would seem sensible to accept the best compromise by which you have some attacks but avoid too many side-effects from your medication. The need to limit treatment to a level that can prevent, for example, major tonic-clonic seizures and restrict the number of more seizures to an acceptable level,

while avoiding your having to walk around in a zombie-like
state, needs to be discussed and fully understood both by you
and your doctor.

Should you stop treatment?

Doctors treating epilepsy have very clear ideas about beginning and continuing therapy, but, perhaps, less often consider
stopping treatment or limiting the amount of medication
used. These possibilities are very important to people with
epilepsy. As many as 70 to 80 per cent of people with epilepsy
will stop having seizures very soon after they begin treatment.
Should they continue to take drugs for the rest of their lives,
thereby running the risk of side-effects, or should they be
advised to stop their treatment?

It is usual to continue treatment for at least two to three
years before considering this. Even then the question is very
difficult to answer. We know that approximately 20 per cent
of people who develop epilepsy during childhood and
approximately 40 per cent of those who develop it during
adult life will have further seizures if medication is stopped
after a two to three year period free of attacks. The people
who are likely to be at greatest risk of suffering further
seizures if they stop taking drugs are:

- those whose epilepsy is related to an identified cause
- those whose epilepsy has been difficult to control in the
  past
- those with juvenile myoclonic epilepsy

Before any decision is made to withdraw drugs, you and
your doctor should discuss all the risks and possible benefits
of this action. Perhaps the most important factor in reaching a
decision is your own attitude. Some people feel very insecure
at the thought of stopping their treatment, others that taking
medication is inherently bad and treatment should be avoided
if at all possible. On the one hand, drivers have to take the
risks of further seizures most seriously; in the UK a single
seizure after stopping treatment will result in the loss of your
driving licence for at least 12 months. On the other hand,
women should consider a trial of drug withdrawal before

pregnancy so as to have the best chance of a pregnancy free from drugs and seizures. Each person has to make his or her own appraisal and decision.

If you are stopping medication
This should be done slowly and gradually; stopping suddenly can produce withdrawal seizures. There are no hard and fast rules about how you do it, but perhaps reducing the medication by a tablet per day at two to four weekly intervals, with the aim of stopping treatment two to three months after you begin the reduction, would be a reasonable approach. In any case, this should be done with your doctor's advice.

Stopping anti-epileptic drugs

Absolute requirement	Factors in favour	Factors against
Minimum of two years fit-free	Childhood epilepsy	Late onset epilepsy
Patient's informed consent	Primary generalized epilepsy	Partial epilepsy
	Idiopathic epilepsy	Symptomatic epilepsy
	Short duration	Long duration
	Normal EEG	Abnormal EEG
	Non-driver	Driver

If you stop your tablets too suddenly and without medical advice you may be more likely to have seizures. Provided you really want to persevere without treatment, it might be worth carrying on – but again, you must talk to your doctor about it. In most circumstances, further seizures on withdrawal mean going back on your previous treatment.

Other kinds of treatment

As we have seen, the fact that someone has epilepsy is not a diagnosis in itself as the condition can have many causes. For this reason people who develop seizures may need other treatments in addition to their anti-epileptic drugs. These range from counselling and psychiatric treatment for people who have been drinking alcohol excessively or taking antibiotics to control infection for people with meningitis or an abscess, to operations for cysts and tumours.

Monitoring treatment

You and your doctor together need to check how your treatment is affecting you. You should give the doctor as much information about yourself as you can. The checklist on page 42 will help you.

People with epilepsy may have regular blood tests to monitor their treatment. For some drugs, phenytoin in particular, there is a range of blood concentrations below which the person might not be receiving the maximum benefit in suppressing seizures and above which there are likely to be side-effects. Although blood tests are unnecessary for most people, they are useful and may be essential for the following:

- people who still have seizures, whose doctors need to decide whether the dose of the drug they are taking can be increased or whether other drugs should be used
- people developing side-effects, particularly if they are taking more than one drug
- special situations, such as pregnancy, liver or kidney failure, or for people who are mentally retarded, when drug intoxication may be difficult to detect
- to check whether a person is taking medication regularly and reliably

Monitoring your Treatment with a Doctor

1. Keep a diary of when seizures occur; their frequency and pattern of occurrence will influence treatment. Seizure diaries are available from hospitals, but any diary can be used.

2. Keep a record of different types of attack and differentiate between them. Minor attacks that do not interfere with your lifestyle need less aggressive treatment than major attacks that do.

3. How do you feel about your medication? Are there any symptoms that you think might be caused by the drugs? Watch out for drowsiness, poor concentration or memory and unsteadiness.

4. Have you had any new symptoms or illnesses since your last visit to the doctor?

5. If seizures have occurred unexpectedly, are there any special circumstances that might be responsible, such as missing your medication, a late night, alcohol?

6. Have you seen any other doctors (perhaps in a hospital casualty department) since your last visit to your regular doctor and have any changes been made to your treatment?

7. Are there any questions about epilepsy that you want your doctor to answer? If so, make a list so you don't forget.

8. Even if you have been very well, ask your doctor to review your treatment every year. Don't simply continue to pick up repeat prescriptions.

Your doctor

People with epilepsy will come into contact with different kinds of doctors during the investigation into their illness. For your continuing treatment you must make sure that only one doctor supervises your checks and medication, and who this is must be clearly understood by everyone concerned. In the UK, for most people who have relatively mild epilepsy, the family doctor is the best person. People with more difficult problems might be put under the supervision of a specialist: a paediatrician for children or a neurologist (a specialist in diseases that affect the nervous system) for older people. In the United States it is usual for the majority to be supervised by their own paediatrician or neurologist.

Specialist advice from a psychiatrist is helpful for people whose mental problems complicate their epilepsy.

Your relationship with your doctor is important. You should feel confident that you can contact him or her when you need to discuss your condition and any worries you may have. You can also ask to be referred to a specialist and you should discuss with your doctor who would be the best person.

Special centres

There are a number of special centres that offer rehabilitation in a carefully controlled environment for people with severe epilepsy *(see page 136)*.

The activities are all those that are aimed at making people more independent. A major part of the work is getting people away from perhaps overprotective family environments. They teach people to make decisions for themselves, get on with new people and form relationships. Basic skills are taught that may be helpful in finding employment. They can also be useful in amending treatments and sorting out diagnoses, and very often they have an important role to play in helping people who have both epilepsy and psychiatric disturbances.

Epilepsy and other medical treatments

You must always inform doctors and dentists about your epilepsy when seeing them for other conditions. Your dentist, for example, will need to know if you are taking phenytoin, which can cause swelling of the gums. Your epilepsy or your medication might also influence whether you receive treatment in the dentist's surgery or in a local dental hospital.

Surgery

Operations to control epilepsy are possible for some people for whom drugs have proved unsuccessful. Two different kinds of approaches are used. Most commonly an operation aims to remove that part of the brain where the seizures begin. Such an operation usually removes part of the temporal lobe, but some operations can be made on other parts of the brain as long as there is no risk to the individual's physical and mental well-being. A second type of operation does not remove any of the brain but divides the connections between various parts of the brain (callosotomy or multiple subpial resection). The second kind of operation is much more rarely done.

There are relatively few operations performed for epilepsy in the United Kingdom, but this kind of treatment is becoming more widely available in specialist centres in the UK and is much more commonly used in the United States. As many as 50–70 per cent of people who have operations for epilepsy can be cured, whilst perhaps another 10–25 per cent are very much improved. The success of the operation are never, however, 100 per cent guaranteed and every individual needs to be considered very carefully before a decision to operate is taken.

You may find that it is helpful for you to prepare a written list of questions for the surgeon in advance, as it is easy to forget things that you wanted to discuss at the time. Remember that no two patients are the same and so the discussion with the surgeon will be specific to you and your case. Operations are usually performed soon after the tests have been completed.

Going into hospital

It is important to plan your admission for epilepsy surgery and convalescence quite carefully. In most cases arrangements need to be made at home and at work for a potential period of six to eight weeks when you will be away from your usual duties and responsibilities. It is common during this period of time to feel tired and easily upset. The support of family, friends and colleagues is therefore important at this time. Remember that the operation can be postponed to a later date if work or home circumstances are unfavourable.

It is usual to go into hospital one or two days before surgery to complete the final preparations. This is a opportunity for you to ask the medical and nursing staff any further questions you may have. It is also a good idea to visit the intensive therapy unit (ITU) before your operation, as that is where you will be spending the first night after surgery. The reason for this is to enable the staff to keep a close eye on you during the hours following surgery.

Before the operation

The amount of hair shaved at the time of surgery varies from surgeon to surgeon. Some surgeons still insist on shaving the whole head, whereas some shave only a small strip in the region where the cut is going to be made on your head. This will be shown to you when the procedure is explained. Remember that the hair will quickly regrow. The night before or the morning of the surgery you will need to wash your hair.

You will be visited by an anaesthetist the night before the operation who will discuss your general health with you and explain what the anaesthetic will involve. It is usual for you not to be allowed to eat or drink anything for about six hours before the operation, but you will receive your anti-epileptic medication in the usual way.

Surgery itself takes three to four hours, although the length of each operation does vary according to the type of surgery being carried out.

After the operation

On waking up in the intensive therapy unit, regular pain relief and relief from any nausea are usually given. It is entirely normal to have a headache after surgery but this generally goes during the first couple of days.

It is likely that you will feel tired and sleepy at first. You may have good days and bad days, and this is entirely normal. It is advisable to keep visitors to a minimum for the first three to four days and slowly increase the number after that if you wish.

Seizures may occur within the first week of surgery. They do not mean that the surgery has been a failure. Your medication will need to be checked and possibly adjusted during your stay in hospital. When the staff are happy that you have made an adequate recovery to be discharged, arrangements will be made for you to return home. The length of time that people are kept in hospital after epilepsy surgery does vary and this should be discussed with your doctor.

Recovery from surgery

During the weeks following surgery it is important to take as much rest as possible and avoid stress. Try not to do too much too soon but to gradually increase mental and physical activity. This also applies to returning to work. Some employers are happy for you to start on a part-time basis, perhaps building up over a two to three week period. Before returning to work, discuss your intentions with your doctor or surgeon.

Sexual activity after surgery

The usual advice is that you may resume sexual activity as soon as you wish, provided that you feel mentally and physically ready.

Sport and vigorous exercise after surgery

It is wise to wait until your post-operative check with the surgeon at about six to eight weeks after surgery, then, provided all is well and you feel up to it, you may begin gradually. Building up to the level that you were doing formerly may take a while. It is best not to rush things at first.

Travel after surgery

After the initial weeks of convalescence following surgery, there are no reasons why you should not travel by land or air. However, it is important to remember that you must still be regarded as having epilepsy and therefore when travelling or taking part in recreational activities you must take the same precautions as you would have done prior to surgery, even if you have not experienced seizures following the operation.

Has the surgery been successful?

Before surgery the aim of the operation will have been carefully discussed with you by the surgeon. In many cases, the aim is to stop seizures completely; in others, a reduction in the number or severity of attacks is hoped for. Your medication will probably not be altered for about one year. Whatever the aims of surgery, these will usually have been achieved within two years and surgical follow up discontinued at this point.

It is important to realize, however, that losing seizures must not be expected to solve all life's problems and indeed may lead to other problems and stresses in daily life. It is most important to maintain contact with the hospital and specialist for some time after this period so that any difficulties may be picked up.

It is not unusual to experience a period of depression after epilepsy surgery and if you or your family are concerned about this you should discuss it with the doctor. This often arises because of people's expectations of the person with epilepsy change following surgery when it is successful. They are no longer regarded as being ill and people may become less sympathetic and more impatient. Specialist help is available in cases where the depression goes on for some time or becomes more severe; indeed, treatment for depression is improving all the time.

Other kinds of treatment are used even more rarely. A ketogenic diet, which is rich in fats and oils, is sometimes prescribed for children with bad epilepsy, when drugs have failed. It is by and large unpalatable and difficult to comply with, but it does help in a few cases.

It is safe for people with epilepsy to have surgical treatment for other conditions. Make sure that the surgeon, anaesthetist and medical staff know about your epilepsy and the drugs you take, and continue your regular medication during your stay in hospital.

8

The outlook: cure or control?

One of the most important questions for people who have recently been diagnosed as having epilepsy, and for their families, is can the epilepsy be cured or controlled? The two are obviously different. Cure implies that the medication can be stopped eventually, with no likelihood of further attacks taking place. Control means that attacks may stop, but will probably return if the medication is withdrawn.

The overall outlook, or prognosis, for control and cure is good. Usually attacks can be prevented with drugs and where this is not possible the number of attacks can in most cases be greatly reduced. Between 70 and 80 per cent of people who develop epilepsy will have a long period of remission of seizures, which lasts for many years, and about half of those whose seizures are completely controlled come off their drugs and remain free of attacks. Because virtually everyone who has epilepsy receives treatment with drugs, we cannot be sure whether the cure is a result of this treatment or due to the fact that some kinds of epilepsy occur only at certain ages and people can grow out of them.

Some people continue to have seizures throughout their lives and need lifelong treatment with drugs. Why are these people different from the majority? The following factors seem to influence people's responses to treatment.

Type of seizures and epilepsy

This is probably the most important factor. Partial epilepsies are usually more difficult to control completely – although approximately 50 per cent of people with this kind of epilepsy eventually stop having seizures – and complex partial epilepsy is the most difficult. Although drugs are very effective in preventing tonic-clonic attacks, they are much less effective against more minor partial seizures.

Children with some of the more severe generalized epilepsies, such as infantile spasms and Lennox-Gastaut Syndrome *(see pages 29–30)*, can also be difficult to treat.

The people with the best outlook have an idiopathic generalized epilepsy with a few tonic-clonic seizures without an aura, or true petit mal (typical absence). Ninety per cent of these people stop having attacks after they have been treated and many are able to come off their drugs.

Age of onset

Epilepsy that begins in childhood almost always has a better prognosis than epilepsy that begins later; many childhood epilepsies disappear in adult life. The exception to this is epilepsy that begins in the first year or two of life, often after severe brain damage.

Symptomatic or idiopathic

If the epilepsy is a symptom of brain disease, the chance of complete control is not good. People with brain damage usually have partial seizures or symptomatic generalized epilepsies and both of these have a poor outlook.

These symptomatic epilepsies become more common in later life compared with others. This is probably the reason why age has become an important factor in the prognosis.

Duration and severity

The more frequent and longer the period over which seizures take place, the worse the outlook. For this reason some doctors believe that the sooner a person with epilepsy is treated the better and so they are eager to treat someone who has had only two seizures. Whether this early treatment really does influence the long-term outlook is controversial.

Taking all these factors into account, the best outlook is for children who have had only two or three generalized seizures without an aura and who have no underlying brain disease or damage. The poorest is for older people who have partial seizures that might be a symptom of some brain damage.

Compliance with treatment

One reason for failure to control fits is tablets being taken irregularly! It is important you remember to take your medication as prescribed *(see also page 75–76)*.

Does epilepsy cause brain damage

This is a common misconception. On the whole, people with epilepsy have IQs in the normal range and many are above average. Some people who have suffered brain damage also have epilepsy and might have a learning disability. Then the epilepsy, like the mental retardation, is a result, not a cause, of the brain damage. There are two extremely rare circumstances in which epilepsy can lead to brain damage:

1. Some of the severe childhood epilepsies – infantile spasms and Lennox-Gastaut Syndrome *(see pages 29, 30)* – can rarely occur in otherwise normal infants. These children may develop brain damage if the epilepsy is not controlled.
2. Brain damage can be caused by status epilepticus. The risk is greatest to children having prolonged febrile convulsions *(see page 36)*. This is because the brain cells may become so overactive that the blood cannot transport enough oxygen to the brain to keep up with it and so brain cells die.

Status epilepticus is a condition in which one tonic-clonic seizure succeeds another without the person regaining consciousness. When this continues for more than 20 minutes or half an hour it becomes potentially dangerous, threatening brain damage. The commonest reason why this happens to people who already have epilepsy is that they have stopped their drug treatment very suddenly.

9

Research

Our understanding of, and ability to treat, epilepsy have improved dramatically in the last 100 years. At present the speed of advance is increasing and although epilepsy is not a condition for which there is ever likely to be a sudden breakthrough that will produce a cure for everyone, we are optimistic that the outlook for people with epilepsy will improve considerably. Our increased understanding of how drugs are absorbed into the body, how they pass via the blood to the brain to have their action, and how they are broken down and inactivated, has resulted in many improvements in the way older drugs are used. The most obvious result for people with epilepsy has been the introduction of monitoring drug dosages by blood tests.

Over the last 10 years a number of new drugs for the treatment of epilepsy have been introduced and licensed in the United Kingdom. They have all been synthesized by the pharmaceutical industry and tested on animals before undergoing vigorous clinical trials in volunteers. It is increasingly possible to design new compounds to have specific actions on chemicals acting as neurotransmitters that, we would predict, will reduce the likelihood of seizures. As we begin to understand more about the causes of different epilepsies we will increasingly be able to design drugs to correct the underlying abnormality.

Basic research

Many people are concerned about the use of animals and medical research. However, without animal experimentation we would not have gained our understanding of the cellular abnormalities underlying epilepsy and it would not have been possible to develop any of the currently used anti-epileptic drugs. Continuing progress in both these areas is heavily dependent on basic research being undertaken on laboratory animals.

Since the mid-1960s scientists have learnt a great deal more about the way in which neurotransmitters alter the behaviour of nerve cells *(see page 6)*. At present the most exciting area of basic research concerns the neurotransmitters gamma aminobutyric acid (GABA), which has a widespread effect throughout the brain in decreasing the excitability of nerve cells, and glutamate, which increases excitability. Our understanding of the way in which these neurotransmitters are synthesized within nerve cells, stored, released and inactivated has advanced enormously in the last 10 years. We are beginning to recognize that many of the drugs that we use now, and which were discovered by chance, seem to have actions on GABA in the brain that might at least partly explain why they are effective in preventing seizures. We know that a variety of drugs that interfere with GABA in the brain can cause convulsions and it seems that those that increase the activity of GABA can prevent seizures. Drugs have now been developed that increase the actions of GABA in the brain either by imitating it or by preventing its being broken down and thereby activated.

Scientists are also interested in a number of neurotransmitters that increase excitability in the brain, including glutamate and aspartate. Research is beginning into the possibility that excessive activity of these substances might have a role to play in producing epilepsy. Newly developed drugs that interfere with the action of these substances are now being be tested on people for their anti-epileptic actions. While a lot of basic research is done on animals, all drugs must eventually be tested and found to be effective and safe for human beings. People with epilepsy can be directly involved in research by volunteering to take part in trials of new drugs.

There are at present many new drugs at various stages of evaluation. Although the majority will fall by the wayside for one reason or another, some will be found to be effective and safe, and will be approved for use in people with epilepsy. A number of these drugs have been licensed in the UK:

- Vigabatrin (Sabril) prevents the breakdown of GABA in the brain and so helps to prevent epileptic seizures.
- Gabapentin is a drug which has a similar structure to GABA but it is uncertain whether its effect on reducing seizures is due to its effects on GABA.
- Lamotrigine does not appear to work through GABA but it may reduce the action of excitatory neurotransmitters such as glutamate and aspartate. Both these drugs may have advantages in having rather fewer side-effects than some of the drugs previously used to treat epilepsy.
- Topiramate (Topamax) works by a mixture of mechanisms, some of which are like phenytoin and carbamazepine, some of which are via GABA and glutamate. Tiagabine (Gabatril) is a new drug which acts on GABA to prevent its inactivation in the brain.

New investigations

Over the last 50 years the most useful investigation for people with epilepsy has been the EEG. Advancing technology, particularly in electronics, has resulted in the development of telemetry and ambulatory monitoring *(see pages 51–52)*, allowing more prolonged and useful recording. Undoubtedly, these advances will continue and our ability to record the EEG over long periods with relatively little inconvenience to the people being tested will improve.

The most important recent advance in investigation of epilepsy has been magnetic resonance imaging of the brain. Until now CT scanning of the brain has been widely available to produce images of the structure of the brain. However, it does not demonstrate the difference between grey and white matter of the brain very well and it may also fail to show a number of different kinds of scars and tumours of the brain.

Magnetic resonance imaging is a technique that generates images by detecting changes within a powerful magnetic field. This gives remarkable pictures of grey and white matter and identifies a number of different types of brain scar. In particular it can identify damage to the temporal lobes (medial temporal sclerosis) that can be so successfully treated by surgery *(see page 122)*.

Magnetic resonance spectroscopy is also sufficiently adaptable that we can start to measure other things. It is possible to measure changes in blood flow that occur when a part of the brain is used for a particular function, such as moving a hand or arm. This kind of functional imaging may become more important in the investigation of people with epilepsy and in planning surgical treatment. Magnetic resonance technology can also allow the estimation of the concentration of a number of chemicals in the brain, including neurotransmitters. This may again prove to be a useful and important 'non-invasive' way of examining brain function.

Other techniques can similarly create images of the functioning of the brain. One such technique is positron emission tomography (PET scanning).

For this test isotopes emitting positrons are injected into a blood vessel or inhaled. Low levels of radiation, which are no risk to the person being tested, are emitted by the isotope. These can be detected by special instruments. The data are then processed by computer to produce a picture that shows areas of high, or low, brain activity. The isotopes used are those of sugars or oxygen, which are taken up most by the most active areas of the brain. Trials with PET scanning seem to show that epileptic areas of the brain are less active between fits and more active than the rest of the brain during fits. This test may prove to be helpful in identifying the areas of the brain that are a cause of seizures and so improve the results of operations for the treatment of epilepsy.

A similar but much cheaper technique that is being used to investigate some people with epilepsy is SPECT scanning. This is rather similar to radioactive isotope scanning in which an isotope that emits single photons (a low level of radioactivity) is injected into a vein. This can be used to capture a picture of the blood flow of the brain. As parts of the brain that are damaged and give rise to seizures often have a poor blood supply between seizures and a high blood supply during and immediately after seizures, giving an appropriate isotope may help to pinpoint where fits begin. Because this technique needs only what is called a gamma camera, a machine which is available in many hospitals, research is being undertaken to see whether the use of this simple, cheap technique might simplify investigating people who are being considered for operations for their epilepsy.

Funds for research

It is important to understand how research into epilepsy is funded and what the problems are. Universities and government agencies are important sources of research funds in the United Kingdom. The major grant-giving bodies are the Medical Research Council and the Department of Health. Other large charities also support research (The Wellcome Trust, The Nuffield Foundation, The Wolfson Trust, The Epilepsy Research Foundation). From these sources there is support for research into the basic mechanisms of epilepsy but unfortunately very little money is being spent on research into clinical aspects of epilepsy. A recent survey of the funding of research for neurological disorders in the United Kingdom suggested that if you had a rare condition such as muscular dystrophy, anything up to £250 might be spent on research for every individual with that condition. For people with epilepsy the figure may be as little as 15p per person. It is unfortunately true that the funds available to the Medical Research Council and to universities have been significantly reduced in recent years, making funds for all kinds of medical research more difficult to obtain. It is also unfortunate that, unlike those of other conditions, the epilepsy associations in the United Kingdom make up little of the gap that exists between the needs for research and the funding from the government.

The drug industry is also a vital source of finance for research, and several large drug companies are actively involved in research into epilepsy and the development of new drugs for treating it. It would be very difficult to over-emphasize how important their contribution is. Although drug companies have at times been criticized for making excessive profits, the very stringent regulations that have to be met before a drug can come onto the market and be prescribed mean that drug development is an extremely expensive business. For every new anti-epileptic drug that reaches the market in the next 10 years, many hundreds will have been abandoned during the course of testing and development.

Perhaps most relevant to people with epilepsy and their families is the role played by charities in supporting research. Many large charities support research into brain function in general and epilepsy in particular. You can contribute to the research funds of the national epilepsy associations directly and through fund-raising events, and in this way contribute to advances in the treatment of epilepsy.

USEFUL ADDRESSES

British Isles

Epilepsy Associations

The British Epilepsy Association
Anstey House
40 Hanover Square
Leeds
Yorks. LS3 1BE   Tel: (01532) 439393 for membership, talks
and enquiries; (0345) 089599 National Information Centre

Other branches
72a London St
Reading
Berks. RG1 4SJ   Tel: (01734) 587345

The Old Post-Graduate Centre
Belfast City Hospital
Lisborne Rd
Belfast. BT9 7AB   Tel: (01232) 248414

48 Govan Rd
Glasgow GS1 1JR   Tel: 0141–427 4911

13 Guthrie St
Edinburgh EH1 1JG   Tel: 0131–226 5428

Mersey Region Epilepsy Association
Glaxo Neurological Centre
Norton Street
Liverpool L3 8LR   Tel: 0151–298 2666

Wales Epilepsy Association
Gwynedd Voluntary Services Council

Eldon Square
Dolgellau
Gwynedd   Tel: (01341) 422575

BEA Information Service
(24 hours)

BEA Membership Services	0898 777264
Facts about Epilepsy	0898 777265
Initial Diagnosis	0898 777266
Epilepsy and the Elderly	0898 777267
Epilepsy and the Child	0898 777268
Epilepsy and Driving	0898 777269
First Aid	0898 777270
Medical Management	0898 777271
Epilepsy and Employment	0898 777272
Epilepsy, Sport and Leisure	0898 777273

Callers charged 38p per minute peak rate and 25p per minute
off peak. Callers may leave their names and addresses at the
end of each tape, and literature on the relevant topic will be
posted from the National Information Centre.

Irish Epilepsy Association
249 Crumlin Rd
Dublin W12   Tel: (0001) 516500

Epilepsy Helpline
0345 089599 (cost of local call)
9a.m.–4.30p.m. Mon–Thurs
9a.m.–4p.m. Fridays

The National Society for Epilepsy
Chalfont Centre
Chalfont St. Peter
Gerrards Cross
Bucks. SL9 0RJ   Tel: (01494) 873991
Epilepsy Helpline   Tel: (01494) 601400

Residential Centres for People with Epilepsy
Chalfont Centre for Epilepsy
Chalfont St. Peter
Bucks. SL9 0RJ   Tel: (01494) 873991

David Lewis Centre
Alderley Edge
Cheshire SK9 7UD   Tel: (01565) 872613

Meath Home for Women and Girls with Epilepsy
Westbrook Road
Godalming
Surrey GU7 2QJ   Tel: (01486) 85095

The Maghull Homes
The Bartlett Home
Liverpool Road South
Maghull
Merseyside L31 8BR   Tel: 0151–526 4133

Quarrier's Homes
Bridge of Weir
Renfrewshire PA11 3SA   Tel: (01505) 612224

St. Elizabeth's School
Much Hadham
Herts. SG10 6EW   Tel: (01279) 843451

Assessment Centres for Epilepsy
Bootham Park Hospital
Bootham
York YO3 7BY   Tel: (01904) 54664

Chalfont Centre for Epilepsy
Chalfont St. Peter
Bucks. SL9 0RJ   Tel: (01240) 73991

David Lewis Centre*
Alderley Edge
Cheshire SK9 7UD   Tel: (01565) 872613

Maudsley Hospital, Epilepsy Unit*
Denmark Hill
London SE5 8AZ   Tel: 0171–703 6333

* Not designated as a special assessment centre but provides an assessment facility.

Park Hospital for Children
Old Road
Headington
Oxford OX3 7LQ   Tel: (01865) 245651

Schools for Children with Epilepsy
Lingfield Hospital School
St. Piers Lane
Lingfield
Surrey RH7 6PN

St. Elizabeth's School
South End
Much Hadham
Herts. SG10 6EW

The David Lewis Centre
Warford
Alderly Edge
Cheshire SK9 7UD

Special bracelets or pendants
SOS Talisman
212–220 Regent's Park Road
London N3 3HP

Medic-Alert Foundation
11/13 Clifton Terrace
London N4 3JP

Useful Contacts and Further Reading
BREAK – Holiday Club for Disabled People
Tel: (01263) 823170

British Sports Association for the Disabled
Tel: 0171–490 4919

GLAD – Greater London Association for the Disabled
London Disability Guide   Tel: 0171–274 0107

Jubilee Sailing Trust   Tel: (01703) 631388

Physically Disabled and Able Bodied (PHAB)
12–14 London Road
Croydon CR0 2TA   Tel: 0181–668 1612

Ticket Scheme
Cheap tickets to theatres, galleries, shows, cinema, etc.
Tel: 0171–700 0100/8138

Royal Association for Disability and Rehabilitation (RADAR)
25 Mortimer Street
London W1N 8AB   Tel: 0171–250 3222

Australia

National Epilepsy Association of Australia
Mr Robert Gourley
Executive Director
PO Box 554
Lilydale, Vic 3140

Epilepsy Association of the Australian Capital Territory Inc.
Shout Office
Hughes Community Centre
Wisdom Street
Hughes, ACT 2605

Epilepsy Association of New South Wales
468 Pennant Hills Road
Pennant Hills, NSW 2120
PO Box 521
Pennant Hills, NSW 2120

Epilepsy Association of Queensland
Room 438
Penney's Building
210 Queen Street
Brisbane, Qld 4000

Epilepsy Association of South Australia Inc.
471 Regency Road
Prospect, SA 5082
PO Box 596
Prospect East, SA 5082

Epilepsy Association of Tasmania Inc.
86 Hampden Road
Battery Point
Hobart, Tas 7000
PO Box 421
Sandy Bay, Tas 7005

Epilepsy Association of Victoria
818–822 Burke Road
Camberwell, Vic 3124

West Australian Epilepsy Association (Inc.)
14 Bagot Road
Subiaco, WA 6008

INDEX

ACUPUNCTURE

An introductory guide to the technique and its benefits

Michael Nightingale

Acupuncture is internationally recognised and respected as a powerful and effective healing technique. It is part of a complete system of medicine which has been practiced in China for many thousands of years, and consists of inserting very fine needles into the skin at certain points to correct imbalances within the body, which can lead to disease or discomfort.

Michael Nightingale explains the philosophy behind the technique and gives an informative and reassuring introduction to the treatment, explaining which conditions are particularly suited to treatment by acupuncture and alternative methods of treatment, such as using lasers or massage instead of needles.

T'AI CHI

The essential introductory guide

Alan Peck

T'ai Chi is an ancient Chinese martial art, instantly recognizable for its slow, graceful movements. In the introduction, Alan Peck explains how T'ai Chi teaches a flexible and yielding response to confrontation and the physical, mental and spiritual benefits practising T'ai Chi can bring to our daily lives.

Packed with practical information on finding a class, basic exercises and techniques as well as being illustrated with line drawings which enable the novice to experiment with the feel of T'ai Chi, this book is ideal both for beginners and advanced students, for whom it explains how to progress further with T'ai Chi, the higher states, and how often you should practice.

SHIATSU

An introductory guide to the technique and its benefits

Ray Ridolfi

Shiatsu is a Japanese word meaning 'finger pressure' and is sometimes referred to in the West as 'acupressure'. Like acupuncture and aromatherapy, shiatsu aims to balance the body's energies and it works on the principle that healing touch can trigger self-healing in the patient. It has been effectively used in Eastern medicine for several thousand years.

In this book Ray Ridolfi explains what to expect from a course of treatment, and gives specific advice on types of condition that can benefit from shiatsu. This straightforward guide answers all your questions about shiatsu as well as providing background information on this increasingly popular treatment.

THE STRESS AND RELAXATION HANDBOOK

A practical guide to self-help techniques

Jane Madders

In this informative book, Jane Madders, who taught stress management for over 40 years, describes numerous relaxation techniques which can help everyone to counteract stress and lead a healthier life.

Fully illustrated throughout, the book guides you through relaxation exercises which you can apply during everyday activities such as walking or while at work, as well as techniques specially designed for parents, children and older people. There are also exercises to help manage the kind of pain and tension found in problems such as migraine, insomnia, period pain and digestive disorders.

To order your copy direct from Vermilion (p&p free) use the form below or call TBS DIRECT on **01621 819596**.

Please send me

...... copies of **ACUPUNCTURE** @ £6.99 each

...... copies of **T'AI CHI** @ £6.99 each

...... copies of **SHIATSU** @ £5.99 each

...... copies of **THE STRESS AND RELAXATION**
                      HANDBOOK @ £8.99 each

Mr/Ms/Mrs/Miss/Other (BlockLetters)

Name..

....

Address..

....

....

Postcode...............................Signed.....................................

HOW TO PAY

☐ I enclose a cheque/postal order for £............................
made payable to 'TBS The Book Services Ltd'.

☐ I wish to pay by Access/Visa/Switch/Delta card
(delete where appropriate)

Card Number ☐☐☐☐☐☐☐☐☐☐☐☐☐☐☐☐

Expiry Date ☐☐☐☐

Post order to **TBS Direct, TBS The Book Service Ltd, St. Lukes Chase, Tiptree, Essex, CO5 0SR.**

POSTAGE AND PACKING ARE FREE. Offer open in Great Britain including Northern Ireland. Books should arrive less than 28 days after we receive your order; subject to availability at time of ordering. If not entirely satisfied return in the same packaging and condition as received with a covering letter within 7 days. Vermilion books are available from all good booksellers.